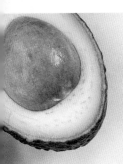

RISE & SHINE

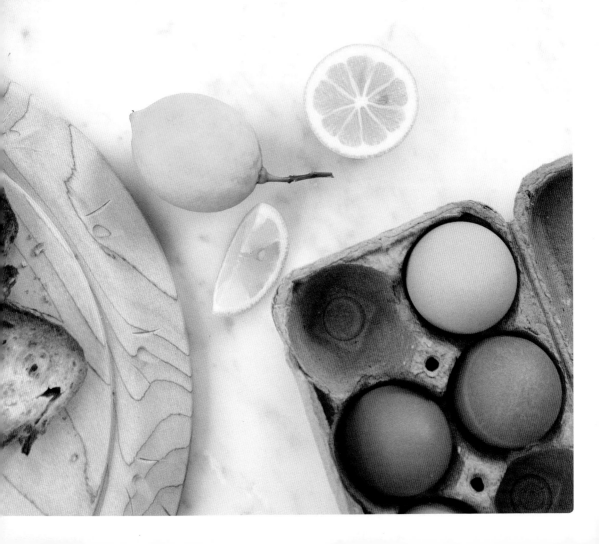

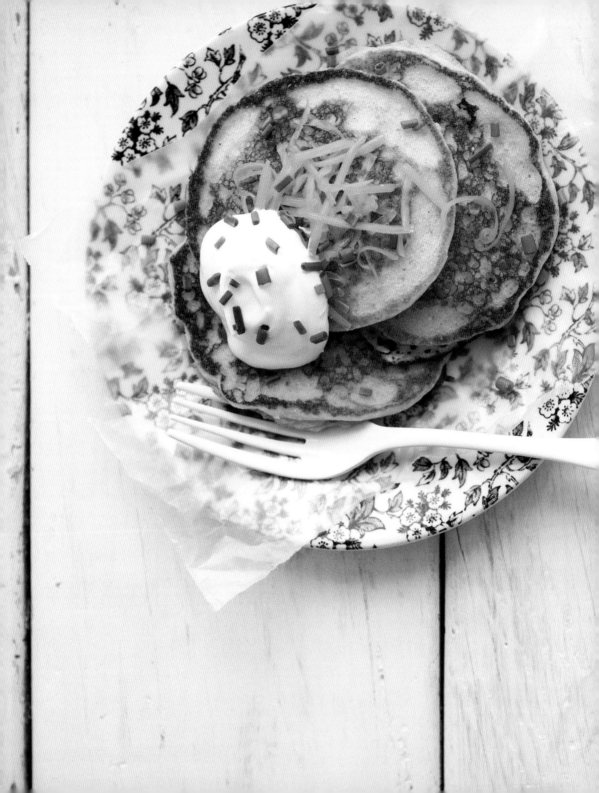

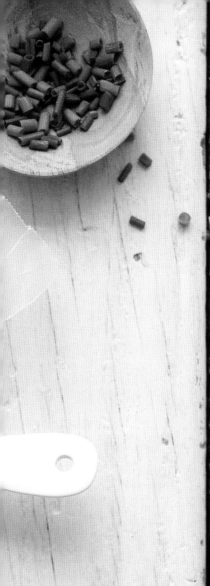

RISE & SHINE

BETTER BREAKFASTS
for BUSY MORNINGS

· · · ·

KATIE SULLIVAN MORFORD

PHOTOGRAPHS BY ERIN SCOTT

Ⓡℬ

ROOST BOOKS
BOULDER
2016

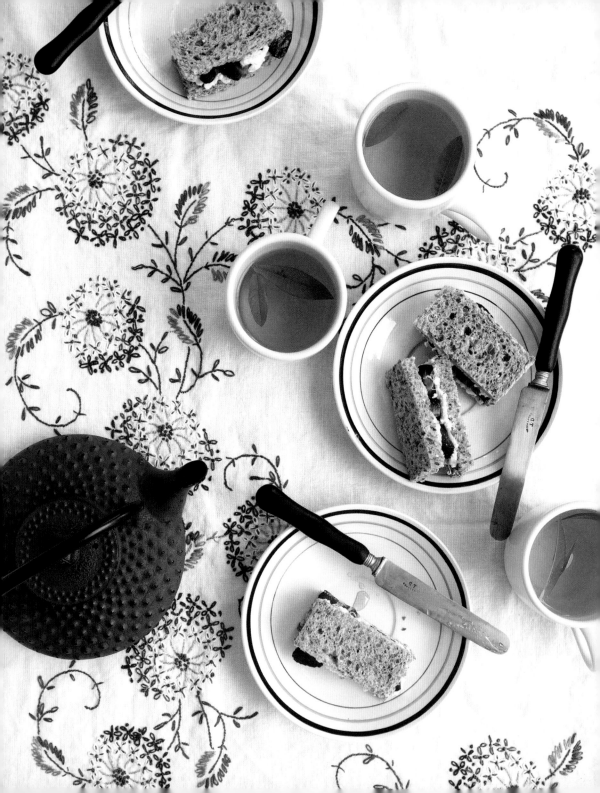

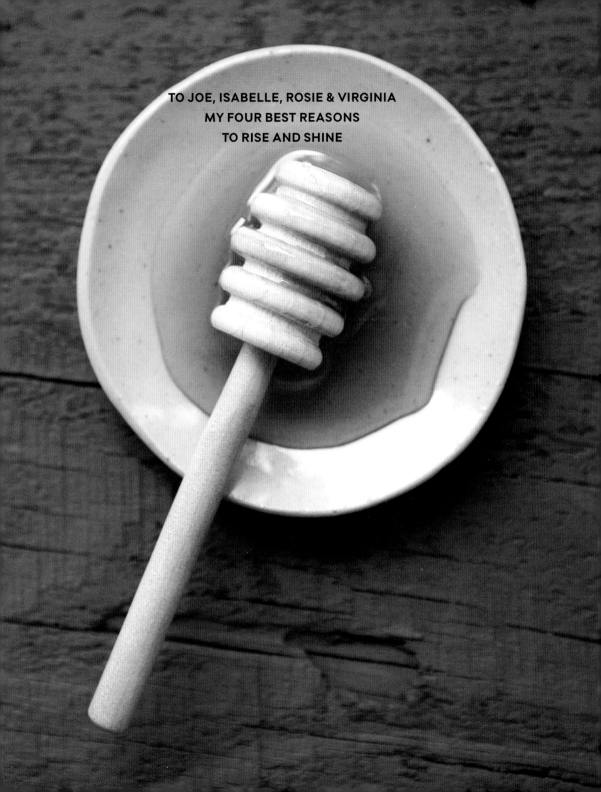

TO JOE, ISABELLE, ROSIE & VIRGINIA
MY FOUR BEST REASONS
TO RISE AND SHINE

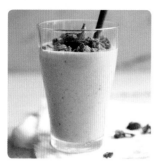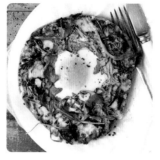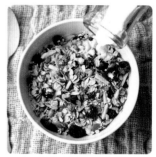

CONTENTS

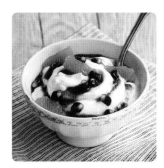
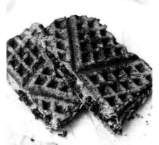
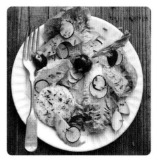

CONTENTS

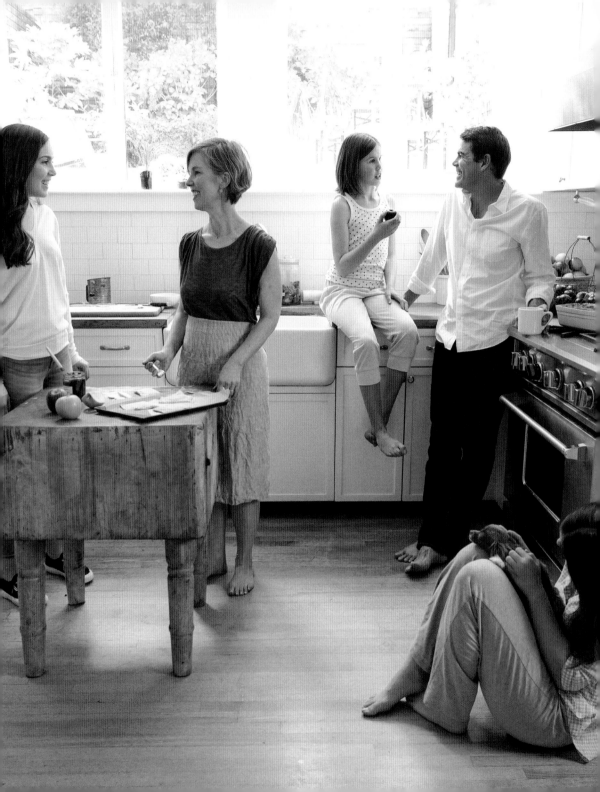

INTRODUCTION

since my kids were tiny, I've begun many mornings with a little ritual that involves poking my head into their bedrooms and whispering, "Rise and shine . . . ," just loud enough to wake them from their sleep. It's exactly how my own mom roused my siblings and me when we were growing up, a practice that starts the day off on a note hopeful enough to coax children from the comfort of warm beds.

But this gentle waking is often (usually?) followed by chaos. So much needs to happen between sleep and the start of the school day. There are showers to take, beds to make, outfits to choose, shoes to tie, backpacks to fill, lunches to pack, and teeth to brush. And this is just the practical side of the story. It doesn't even take into account the child who won't get up, the one who must be prodded along every step of the routine, the one having a bad hair day or a "wrong side of the bed" day. And then there is all that needs to happen for parents, some of whom have been up half the night with a baby or working into the wee hours for a boss who doesn't care that they have a family to get out the door.

As a result, what should be the priority of the morning—breakfast—becomes an afterthought. The meal we all hear is the most important of the day, especially for kids, becomes a "flying by the seat of our pants" postscript. It's reduced to shoveling in a few bites of Cheerios while pulling on winter coats, scarfing down a cereal bar en route to the bus, sometimes, or eating nothing at all.

This book is the answer to every parent who has struggled to get breakfast on the table—and to get their child to actually eat it. It comes from my personal experience

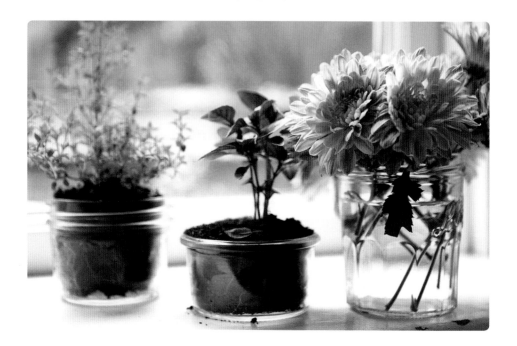

in making family meals for the past seventeen years, a job I've managed without relying heavily on the beguiling lineup of supermarket convenience foods.

Inside this book you'll find recipes for seventy-five breakfast favorites, most of which are entry-level easy, with a generous number requiring no more than five to ten minutes of hands-on time. You'll also discover many dishes that can be made ahead, so the only requirement for eating breakfast in the morning is, well, to eat breakfast. The recipes draw on my expertise as both a registered dietitian and a culinary professional, which means they balance good nutrition with good taste. Every last one was rigorously vetted by my own team of in-house critics—otherwise known as my children—and then tested by a small army of parent and teen recipe testers.

In the process of writing this book, nearly everyone I spoke to responded the same way: with an enthusiastic "I LOOOOVE breakfast." Yet, many of these same folks confessed that breakfast often gets the shaft. This book intends to change that. It honors our passion for the first meal of the day by arming you with recipes and inspiration for those 260 week-day mornings a year that can make or break a healthful diet. The aim, ultimately, is to give you and your kids something to really "rise and shine" about. Breakfast!

1

WHY MORNING MATTERS

whether or not breakfast truly is the most important meal of the day is up for debate. I'd argue that all meals matter because, collectively, they form the balance of our diet: the good, the bad, and the ugly. What's unique about breakfast, though, is that by the time morning arrives, most of us have been without a bite to eat for somewhere in the neighborhood of twelve hours. It makes sense that our bodies need refueling, particularly children, who have smaller tanks that need to be topped off regularly.

There is plenty of research demonstrating the upside of getting breakfast under your belt, particularly where kids are concerned. Studies have found that children and teens who take in a morning meal tend to do better in school through improved memory, ability to concentrate, and better test grades. Kids also benefit socially, due to improved mood and better social interactions with teachers and classmates. In addition, eating breakfast is linked with lower body weight and less weight gain over time. Among children and adolescents, breakfast eaters have been shown to be less likely to be overweight, while breakfast skippers are at higher risk for being overweight or obese.

Let's not forget something a little less measurable but no less important: breakfast is an opportunity for family time—to sit across the table from one another over a bowl of oatmeal or to stand at the stove together and scramble a pan of eggs. Between busy school and work schedules, the morning may be the only quality time your family has all day.

So yes, breakfast does matter, but here's the rub: not all meals are created equal.

WHAT MAKES A GOOD BREAKFAST?

Great question. What, really, does a balanced breakfast look like? Recently, a group of nutrition experts gathered research and put their heads together to decide just that. In a nutshell, they concluded that breakfast should:

- Make up 15 to 25 percent of daily calories from a combination of carbohydrates, protein, and healthy fats.
- Feature sensible portions based on age, gender, and daily energy needs.
- Make a generous dent in our daily nutrient requirements, with a goal of at least 20 percent for as many nutrients as possible.
- Emphasize nutrient-dense foods—that is, foods that pack in a lot of nutrition for the amount of calories delivered.
- Ideally, be made up of at least three of the food groups—that is, grains, fruits, vegetables, protein foods, and dairy foods.

I appreciate the data, but when it comes to feeding my family, I think less about calories, percentages, and grams of fat and more about the food itself, focusing on those three (or more) food groups we're aiming for. I figure, if we fill our plates with a variety of whole foods, eat when we're hungry, and stop when we've had enough, the rest will usually take care of itself. With that in mind, here's what I focus on, nutrition-wise, when it comes to setting the breakfast table.

MORE FRUITS AND VEGETABLES

Most of us fall well short of eating enough fruits and vegetables, kids included. Me included. Consider the fact that the USDA recommends half of our plates be filled with them. Realistically, how often does that happen? To come within striking distance, we can't overlook the chance breakfast gives us to add something from the produce aisle, whether it's adding leftover broccoli to scrambled eggs or topping cold cereal with raspberries. When it comes to picking your produce, variety counts too. Aim to eat with the seasons so that over the course of the calendar year, you've packed your plate with the full rainbow. And don't discount the freezer section of the market, because nutritionally, frozen fruits and vegetables stack up well against fresh, and they can be handy, particularly between seasons when choices aren't so abundant. As for organics, choose pesticide-free produce if you can swing it. That said, what matters, first and foremost, is getting in plenty of fruits and vegetables. If the economics of buying organic is a barrier, put your organic food dollars toward what has become known as the "dirty dozen"—produce known to have the highest pesticide residues:

THE DIRTY DOZEN

1. Apples 2. Peaches 3. Nectarines 4. Strawberries 5. Grapes
6. Celery 7. Spinach 8. Bell peppers 9. Cucumbers
10. Cherry tomatoes 11. Imported snap peas 12. Potatoes
(Source: Environmental Working Group)

LESS RELIANCE ON PACKAGED FOOD

Let's be honest: I'm not at home bottling milk from backyard goats or grinding grains for home-baked bread. I'm a busy mom, and just like most other parents, I include convenience foods in my shopping cart. That said, I aim for fewer packaged goods and with fewer ingredients, avoiding what's artificial, super-sugary, or hyperprocessed. If I can pull together a breakfast that's mostly homemade, it ups the likelihood that it will also be nourishing, delicious, and, most important, eaten. It also means I get to choose the ingredients that go into my food, which results in less environmental waste through less packaging.

CARBOHYDRATES THAT COUNT

Carbs are bad, right? That may be what the latest diet book or skinniest celebrity would have you believe, but carbohydrate-rich foods are in fact very good and an important part of a balanced diet. What's confusing is that carbohydrates show up in everything from squishy white bread and "sugar cereal" to quinoa and whole grain farro. Same nutrient, different package. The key is to reach for less-processed carbohydrate-rich foods, such as *whole grain rye bread, steel-cut oatmeal, rolled oats, corn tortillas, polenta, brown rice,* and *barley,* to name just a few. These are slow-release carbs, meaning they provide more sustained energy than heavily processed ones. This is something that's particularly important at breakfast, when we need quick energy (which all carbohydrates provide) but don't want to bottom out an hour into the morning. In our house, it's not all whole grains all the time, but I do my best to stock more quality carbs than not. If brown rice and whole wheat bread aren't part of your repertoire, don't fret. Shifting to a more whole grain focus doesn't need to happen overnight; it can occur organically and gradually over time. Baby steps.

PLENTY OF PROTEIN

It can be easy to let breakfast pass us by without getting protein in there. I myself am a reformed toast-for-breakfast eater and have had more than a few meals of cold cereal in a cup, hold the milk. The missing piece, among other nutrients, was protein—the smear of nut butter on bread or the cold milk over cereal. Protein has the potential to help steady our blood sugar, deliver key nutrients, and keep us satiated in a way that carbo-hydrates alone do not. Breakfast-friendly protein sources are many, including *eggs, yo-gurt, milk, soy milk, kefir, cottage cheese and other cheeses, tofu, nuts, seeds, nut butter and peanut butter, beans, smoked fish,* and *ham.* It's not hard to work these foods into breakfast, from topping oatmeal with chopped nuts to downing a glass of milk alongside a slice of homemade banana bread.

AN EYE ON CALCIUM

Many of us (most notably, adolescent girls) are falling short of getting enough calcium in our diet. This mineral, along with its "helper" nutrient, vitamin D, is essential for healthy bones, and I can think of no better meal in which to up your intake than break-fast. Milk and yogurt are morning staples. And if you can't do dairy, most plant-based milks are fortified with just as much calcium as cow's milk, and sometimes more. Other calcium sources for breakfast include *cheese, calcium-fortified soy milk, kefir, almonds* and almond butter, blackstrap molasses, tahini, calcium-fortified cereals, tofu (made with calcium-sulfate), and dark leafy greens, such as kale and collards.

AN EMPHASIS ON HEALTHY FATS

It wasn't long ago that we all seemed to be terrified of dietary fat. Egg-white omelets and fat-free cookies were very much in vogue. The thinking has shifted, though, as we now recognize the importance of fat in health and disease prevention. From a practical standpoint, fat can play a role in staving off hunger because it takes longer to digest than other nutrients. Translation: Top half of a bagel with sliced avocado, and it may sustain you better than a whole bagel, for about the same number of calories. The key is to aim for foods rich in healthier fats—olive oil, nuts, seeds, nut butter, salmon, and avocado—and put less emphasis on foods high in unhealthy fats—sausage, fatty cuts of beef and pork, palm oil, and large amounts of cheese. Foods high in omega-3 fats, such as salmon, sardines, walnuts, and flaxseeds, earn bonus points because they're linked to a whole host of health benefits.

EASY ON THE OJ

How orange juice became the official drink of the American breakfast is a complicated tale that has more to do with good marketing than good nutrition, as far as I can gather. Truth? I'm not a big fan. Are there bigger fish to fry than ousting the simple glass of OJ? Sure. And do I occasionally include it on our breakfast table? Yes. But for most meals, I'd rather have everyone fill up on whole fruit than juice. The natural sugar and calories in juice are more concentrated than in fruit. Plus, juice lacks whole fruit's fiber, which is so important for healthy digestion, among other benefits. For hydrating kids in the morning, I recommend good old-fashioned water, milk, or if you want to get fancy, herbal tea. If drinking your morning orange juice is nonnegotiable, stock up on small juice glasses and aim to limit your portion to four ounces or so.

LESS SWEET STUFF

Sweetness appears to be the resounding theme in much of what we traditionally think of as breakfast food. It's our early-morning crutch. Consider how big a role added sugar plays

REMODEL YOUR BREAKFAST

Making just a few adjustments to basic breakfasts can have a significant impact on nutritional value. Have a peek:

TRADITIONAL VERSION	THE REMODEL	BENEFITS
Cup of strawberry yogurt	Plain yogurt with strawberries and My Girls' Granola (page 66) or Apricot Ginger Cluster Granola (page 69)	More protein, less refined sugar, more nutrients, more fiber
Plain bagel with cream Cheese	Half of a whole grain bagel with avocado and sliced egg	More protein, more fiber, more vitamin E, more iron
Frosted Flakes cereal with milk	Whole grain cereal with sliced banana, toasted almonds, and milk	Less sugar, more protein, more potassium, more fiber
Scrambled eggs on buttered white toast	Veggie Scramble Pita Pockets (page 56)	More vitamins and minerals, more antioxidants, more fiber
Instant oatmeal packet with a glass of orange juice	Homemade "Better Than Boxed" Instant Oatmeal (page 77) with a glass of milk	Less sugar, more protein, more calcium, less dramatic rise and drop in blood sugar

in the following morning staples, particularly when procured at a supermarket or coffee shop: pastries, sweet rolls, cereal bars, fruit-flavored yogurt, donuts, breakfast cereal, muffins, instant oatmeal, smoothies, coffee drinks, and pancakes, waffles, and French toast covered in pancake syrup. A cinnamon roll can have upwards of ¼ cup of sugar in a single bun. As a result, many of us are starting the day with a sugar high, likely to be followed by a blood sugar and energy crash. Not ideal. That said, I do enjoy the likes of muffins, quick breads, and pancakes in the morning, and there's no shortage of baked goods in this book. The aim is to make sure these foods are delivered in an otherwise nourishing package, in a reasonable portion, and not every single day of the week. It's about balance and moderation.

BUYER'S GUIDE TO BETTER BASICS

Now that we know the essentials of a balanced breakfast, let's break it down further and talk ingredients. Anytime you start to look at food under a microscope, it can all start sounding a little complicated, so please take these suggestions with a grain of salt and tailor them to suit your needs. You know better than anyone about your family, your budget, and what is available where you live and shop.

EGGS

It seems like you might need a degree in animal husbandry to decipher the label on an egg carton. If you're wondering what it all means, the following definitions should help. Keep in mind, there is room for interpretation here. Two organic egg farms may look the same on paper but be worlds apart in actuality. For my own family, I typically buy organic eggs, but sometimes I reach for eggs pasteurized in the shell, particularly for recipes that call for undercooked or raw eggs. Once in a while, when I'm at the farmers' market and dazzled by a carton of pretty little blue- or green-hued pasture-raised eggs, I'll spend the extra money and relish every one.

Organic—Eggs are laid by cage-free hens raised on organic feed and without antibiotics. Hens are allowed access to the outdoors with unlimited access to water.

Free Range—This simply indicates that the hens have access to the outdoors for at least part of the day and are not housed in enclosures.

Cage-Free—The hens are not caged, are housed indoors, and have unlimited access to fresh food and water.

Pasture-Raised or Pastured—No government-regulated labeling standard exists, but the suggestion is that hens roam free outdoors to forage on their natural diet of plants and insects with some feed supplementation.

Pasteurized—Eggs are gently heated to kill salmonella and other pathogens, making them safe to eat undercooked or raw.

Omega-3—The hens' diets are supplemented with omega-3–rich foods, making the eggs significantly higher in these fatty acids.

Vegetarian—The hens are fed a vegetarian diet (by the way, chickens are omnivores by nature, not vegetarians).

Hormone-Free—These labels are meaningless, because hormones aren't used for hens laying eggs for human consumption.

Antibiotic-Free—This is an assurance that the hens were not given antibiotics. However, it is worth noting that antibiotics aren't routinely used in the egg industry, and when they are, it's typically for treating sick hens. Even so, the probability of antibiotic residues in eggs is extremely low.

BREAD

So many varieties line the supermarket bread section, it can be tricky to figure out the best of the bunch. Look past what is often marketing hype on the front of the package to the Nutrition Facts label on the back. The most nutritious loaves are the ones that feature a whole grain—such as "whole wheat" or "whole oats"—as the first ingredient. This means the bran and germ, the primary sources of fiber and nutrients, haven't been processed out of the flour. Steer clear of breads with a laundry list of additives and preservatives, high-fructose corn syrup, and coloring. If you have a bakery within easy reach, check out what they have to offer, because they're likely to use fairly pure ingredients. They may even have a bread slicer to cut loaves into toaster-ready slices. Last, consider making your own; the No-Knead Brown Bread on page 174 is a terrific place to start.

YOGURT

At its best, yogurt is delicious, nourishing, and immensely versatile. At its worst, it's more akin to junk food than health food. Here's what to look for when considering your options in the dairy aisle.

Less Sugar: One 6-ounce container of unsweetened low-fat yogurt has roughly 12 grams of naturally occurring sugar from the lactose in the milk. But manufacturers often get busy with the sugar shaker and really pile it on. Compare various brands and find one with less added sugar. Or better yet, buy plain yogurt and dress it up in your own kitchen, using fruit, honey, preserves, and the like. Alternatively, mix equal parts plain and fruit yogurt; you'll immediately cut the added sugar in half.

No Artificial Sweeteners: Keep an eye out for yogurt labeled "light"—that's often code for aspartame, acesulfame-K, and other artificial sweeteners. Chemicals are for chemists, not kids.

Fewer Additives: Call me old-fashioned, but I like yogurt with straightforward ingredients: milk, yogurt cultures, and little else. Unfortunately, many brands pad their products with artificial colors and flavors, stabilizers, and thickeners. My rule of thumb? Less is more.

MILK

Buying a carton of milk used to be dreamily uncomplicated: it was simply a matter of choosing between fat-free, low-fat, and whole. Nowadays, the options seem endless, with the expansion into organic, grass-fed, lactose-free, goat, and numerous plant-based options. In our house, 1% organic cow's milk is the refrigerator staple. I also often stock a plant-based milk, rotating among almond, soy, and coconut milks. If you're wondering how to sort out the best buy for your family, here are some pros and cons of each.

COW'S MILK

What most Americans have been drinking for generations, cow's milk is minimally processed, naturally high in protein, and a good source of calcium. The ingredients on a carton of most cow's milk include milk and vitamins A and D, and little else. Pretty simple. The downside is that it doesn't go down so well among folks who have a dairy allergy or intolerance. Lactose-free milk is a solution for some, while others can lean on the burgeoning selection of plant milks instead.

SOY MILK

A popular choice for decades, soy milk is nearly as good a protein source as cow's milk. And, although not naturally high in calcium, most soy milk is fortified with it. If concern about GMOs is on your radar, opt for organic soy milk, because the great majority of soy products in this country come from GMO crops. Also, soy milk often has added sweeteners, flavorings, and additives that you may want to skip, so be sure to read the list of ingredients.

NUT, SEED, AND GRAIN MILK

How do you milk an almond? You don't. You just add water, blend the heck out of it, and strain off the liquid. Interest in almond milk, along with hemp, rice, coconut, and other plant milks, has ballooned in the recent past. The pros and cons of these nondairy sources are similar to those of soy milk, with one notable difference: most nut, seed, and grain milk has significantly less protein (less than 1 gram per cup in some cases). So if you're looking to boost protein in breakfast with a glass of milk or bowl of cereal, your rice or almond milk may not be the solution.

SHAKE IT UP

The calcium in almond, soy, and other plant milks can settle at the bottom, so be sure to give the carton a hearty shake before filling your glass.

NUT, SEED, SOY, AND PEANUT BUTTER

Nut butter, and all its various counterparts, is an immensely handy breakfast staple that's cheap, quick, and rich in protein, healthy fats, and other nutrients. With so many options available—almond, peanut, soy, sunflower seed, pumpkin seed, and cashew, among others—there is something for everyone, even those with a nut or peanut allergy. The best buys are the ones containing little more than the nuts, peanuts, or seeds and salt, without any added sugar, hydrogenated oil, or palm oil (the latter two are high in saturated fat). If the oil separation that occurs in natural nut butter bothers you, store it upside down. When you turn the jar over to open it, the solids will be at the top, not the bottom.

READY-TO-EAT CEREAL

We are very much a breakfast-cereal nation, with more than 90 percent of households contributing toward this multibillion-dollar business. No doubt, the convenience of ready-to-eat cereal is hard to beat, but it's wise to be thoughtful about what you buy: many cold cereals pack in as much sugar as you might find in a box of cookies. A good rule of thumb is to aim for a cereal with fewer ingredients, at least 3 grams of fiber, and 5 or fewer grams of sugar per serving. You'll find a list of options that fit the bill on page 79.

ABOUT THE RECIPES
PORTIONS

This is a book for all ages and stages. As such, the recipes include a range of servings intended to cover everyone from the tiniest toddler to the most robust teenager. You're the parent and know your people best, so use your own judgment about the appropriate portion sizes for you and your family.

MEASURING

My aim with this book is for everything to be as unfussy as possible. Why, then, do I have you pull out measuring cups and spoons before your coffee has even had the chance to kick in? I get it. The truth? A fair number of the dishes can be executed successfully without a whole lot of precision. My suggestion is to try a recipe at least one time as written, so you can gauge what you're going for. After that, feel free to ad-lib and make the recipes your own. The exceptions are those that involve baking, as well as pancakes and waffles. For those recipes, accuracy is crucial for success. You'll have the best results if you measure flour and other dry ingredients the way I did when I developed the recipes: by spooning and leveling. Here's how: Rather than plunging a measuring cup into a bag of flour, use a large spoon to scoop flour from the bag into the measuring cup. Then scrape the flat edge of a knife lightly across the top of the cup to level it before adding the flour to the mixing bowl. Easy.

OIL AND BUTTER

I maintain a relatively small pantry of cooking fats in my kitchen. Too many fancy oils, and I start to lose track of what I've got. What you'll find in the recipes are the ones I use the most at home. These include:

Olive Oil: This is my number-one cooking fat, which I prize for its flavor and nutritional properties. Look for extra-virgin oil, an indication that it's less refined, processed without heat or chemical solvents, and higher in antioxidants than other types of olive oil.

Canola Oil: This is a good one for baking because of its mild taste. I look for organic, expeller-pressed canola oil, which indicates the oil is from non-GMO plants grown without pesticides and processed without chemicals or heat.

Grape Seed Oil: Derived from grape seeds left over from wine making, grape seed oil is valued for its neutral flavor, high vitamin E content, and ability to withstand elevated cooking temperatures. "Expeller pressed" on the label means it was processed without heat or chemical solvents.

Butter: Yes, I do love and use butter. It doesn't have the healthy upsides of, say, olive oil, but it does something in cooking that other fats sometimes can't match. I use it thoughtfully and in moderation, with no more than a few tablespoons in any recipe. Because the impact of so little butter on overall saltiness is negligible, in my recipes I usually don't specify salted or unsalted; use what you have in your fridge.

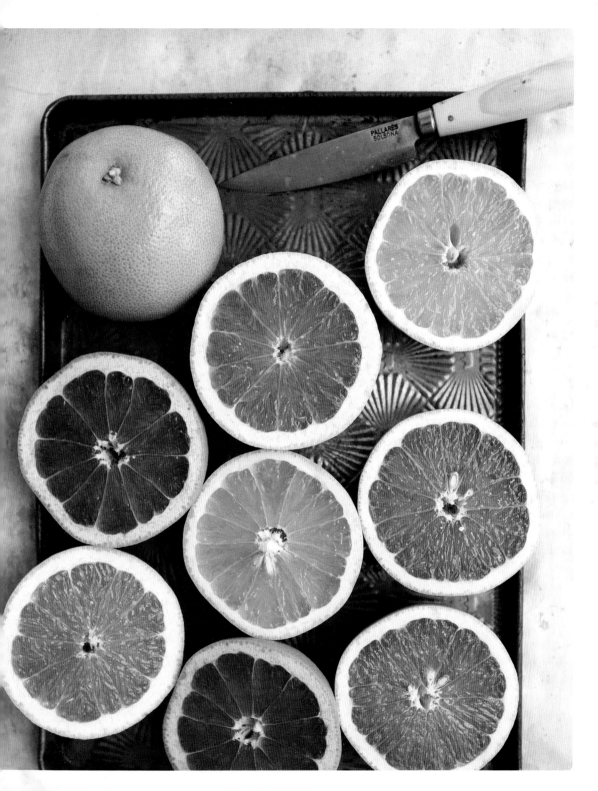

Cooking Oil Spray: I don't use cooking spray often, but I do find it handy for coating hard-to-grease items like muffin tins and the waffle iron. If store-bought cooking spray gives you pause, buy an oil mister online or at a cooking supply store and fill it with oil from your pantry.

FLOURS AND GRAINS

My recipes rely almost entirely on whole grain flours, in part because they're more nutritious, but also because I like what they do for the taste and texture of my food. Whole wheat pastry flour and "white" whole wheat flour are my staples for baked goods, pancakes, and waffles. Both are 100 percent whole grain yet are lighter in texture, milder in flavor, and, in the latter case, paler in color than standard whole wheat flour. Other grains and grain-like foods in my recipes include cornmeal, regular rolled oats (also called old-fashioned oats), steel-cut oats, quinoa, rye flour, brown rice, buckwheat flour, millet, and almond flour. Whole grain flours are more perishable than refined white flour, so if you don't think you'll go through them quickly, store them in the refrigerator or freezer. You can find whole grain flours in the bulk bins or in the baking section of supermarkets, specialty stores, and health food stores. Bob's Red Mill and King Arthur Flour are two reliable sources that offer online sales as well. And, if all else fails, there's always Amazon.com.

SALT

Having experimented with several varieties of salt, I always come back to the generous box of kosher salt as my cooking staple. I pour it into a small box that lives next to the stove. Kosher salt is what I used for the recipes in this book, so if you cook with a finer salt, such as iodized table salt or fine sea salt, you will need to scale back the amount slightly (you can find a conversion chart at www.mortonsalt.com). A few of the recipes also call for a flaky salt, such as Maldon, which is in the "nice to have" category but certainly not a recipe deal breaker.

FAT CONTENT

You'll notice that my recipes don't specify a fat content for cow's milk, yogurt, cottage cheese, and other dairy products. I figure most of you already have your favorites stocked in the fridge, the ones you routinely shop for. I don't see a need for a special trip to the market for low-fat yogurt if you've been happily eating fat-free for decades, nor to buy 1% cow's milk if you have a toddler who drinks only whole. For my own cooking, I generally buy low-fat milk, cottage cheese, yogurt, and sour cream. I sometimes treat myself to whole milk yogurt and always buy full-fat cheese, preferring its richness and flavor. Do what works best for you.

MILK

Most of these recipes were developed using cow's milk, and where the type of milk isn't specified in a recipe, cow's milk is assumed. As such, I can't vouch for how recipes will measure up if made with soy, almond, or other milk. However, I find smoothies, drinks, grains, and egg dishes work well using plant-based milks, as long as you use an unflavored variety. Where it might get tricky is with baked goods, pancakes, and waffles, because plant milks vary in nutrient profile, viscosity, and sweetness. If a baking recipe calls for a relatively small amount of milk, a swap isn't a big deal, but it may affect the end result.

TAILORING THE RECIPES

In an attempt to help you make the most of my recipes, I've included a series of suggestions for tailoring each one to suit your particular needs. Look for the following tags, and follow their advice as you see fit.

BOOST IT: Ideas for small changes to increase the nutritional value of the recipe. Some of the Boost Its also add to or alter the flavor of a dish.

ADAPT IT: Tips for tweaking recipes to make them more suitable for "adventurous eaters in training." Pint-sized palates sometimes take years to develop to the point where they're ready to embrace eggs with leafy greens or smoothies with a lot of texture.

MAKE AHEAD: Instructions for prepping, wrapping, refrigerating, and/or freezing foods so that in the morning you're well stocked with a meal that's easy to grab and go.

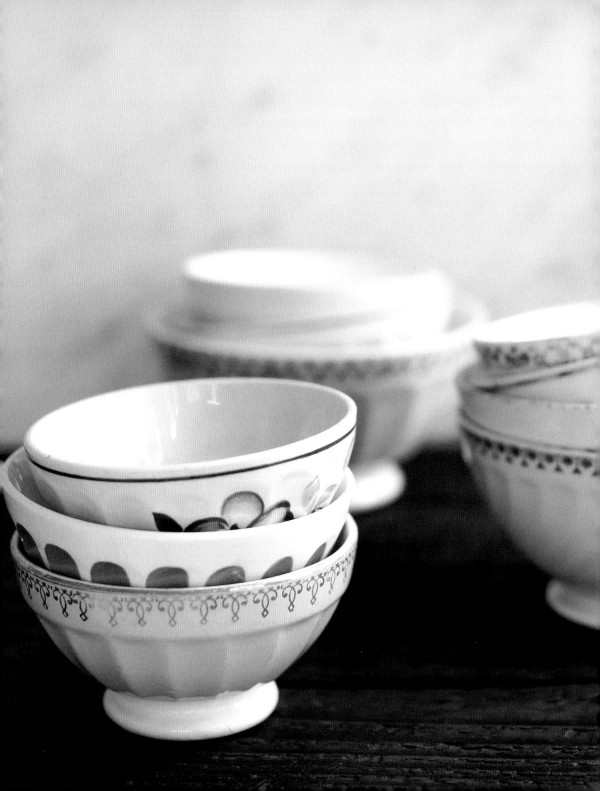

2
MAKING IT HAPPEN

it's one thing to know you want to get a decent breakfast on the table each day, but it's another thing altogether to get the job done. With a bit of forethought, it's not as hard as it may seem, especially if you have a few tips and tricks up your sleeve to help you along the way.

PLANNING

Whether you're an organizational wunderkind or a haphazard home cook, even a smidge of planning can mean the difference between a homemade meal and an emergency pit stop at the drive-through. Here are a handful of tasks you can bang out ahead of time to bring ease to the task of breakfast.

1. GET STOCKED

This is job number one if you want a shot at a good breakfast. But don't worry: stocking up doesn't mean packing the shelves as though you're hibernating for winter. Just a handful of ingredients is all that's required. By way of example, check out how a seven-item grocery list translates into five wholesome meals:

Groceries: Yogurt, granola, milk, eggs, berries, spinach, tortillas
Day 1: Yogurt, berry, and granola parfaits
Day 2: Fruit and spinach smoothies
Day 3: Egg and spinach scramble with fruit on the side
Day 4: Granola with milk and berries
Day 5: Egg and spinach breakfast burritos

THE BREAKFAST PANTRY

Here's a lineup of breakfast pantry ideas organized by fridge, cupboard, and freezer to get you started:

FRIDGE

Plain yogurt

Milk (cow, soy, and/or other plant-based milk)

Kefir

Eggs

Cream cheese

Cottage cheese

Other favorite cheeses, such as Cheddar, Parmesan, and Monterey Jack

Berries, cut pineapple, cut melon, and other refrigerated fruits

Leafy greens (to toss into eggs or smoothies)

Leftovers (such as rice or vegetables) to be repurposed for breakfast

Smoked salmon

Ham, bacon, or sausage

Made-ahead breakfasts, such as "Get Up and Go" Yogurt Cups (page 90) and Breakfast Baked Apples (page 100)

CUPBOARD AND COUNTERTOP

Seasonal fresh fruit

Dried fruits, such as raisins, dates, and dried apricots

Nuts and seeds

Nut, seed, and/or peanut butter

Oats, both steel-cut and old-fashioned rolled oats

Other breakfast-friendly grains, such as brown rice, quinoa, and polenta

Whole grain breads, pita, and bagels

Whole grain tortillas, such as whole wheat and/or corn

Pancake mix (such as the Rise and Shine Pancake Mix on page 142)

Muesli

Granola

Whole grain breakfast cereal

Whole grain breakfast bars, muffins, and quick breads

FREEZER

Frozen fruit

Peeled bananas (for smoothies)

Spinach, corn, and other freezer-friendly vegetables (to fortify egg dishes)

Yogurt pops

Smoothie cubes (for make-ahead smoothies, see page 38)

Whole grain waffles

Made-ahead breakfasts, such as Freezer-Friendly Breakfast Burritos (page 122) and
    Make-Ahead Mini Spinach Frittatas (page 58)

So, take a minute on a Saturday or Sunday to peruse your pantry and see what's needed, then stop at the market before the week begins.

2. ORGANIZE YOUR GOODS

Think about arranging your breakfast staples in the refrigerator, freezer, and cupboard so that it's handy for you (and your kids) to get at them and get breakfast under way. Little steps can make all the difference, such as having granola in an easy-to-reach jar, making little bags of breakfast trail mix (Good Morning Trail Mix, page 73), or having a bin of sliced fruit at eye level in the fridge.

3. POLL YOUR PEOPLE

Before the week begins, get buy-in from the family about what's on their minds for the morning. Brainstorm. Have them tag along at the market to pick out favorite fruits, raid the bulk bins for hot cereal grains, or choose nuts and dried fruits for making breakfast bars. Get them to help with some of the advanced prep, turning a chore into a family activity.

4. PICK A FEW FOR THE WEEK

You probably don't have the same few dinners day in, day out, so why the same break-fast? Keep it fresh and interesting by mixing it up from week to week. Flip through the recipes in this book and pick out one or two new ones to try every week or so. Variety not only wards off breakfast boredom; it has nutritional upsides as well, because every food provides a different nutrient profile. Consider, for example, how a smoothie on Monday might deliver a hefty serving of fruit, calcium, and vitamin C, while eggs scrambled with grains and greens on Tuesday packs in the protein, B vitamins, and fiber.

5. DO A LITTLE ADVANCED PREP

When you put off all the breakfast preparation to the last minute, it can make for a grumpy morning and leave you with more dishes than you care to clean up. Just a few minutes of prep the night before can make a difference, such as chopping up vegetables from dinner to toss into a breakfast scramble, giving a pot of steel-cut oats a head start, or hard-boiling a few eggs. Even something as simple as setting out your mixing bowl and pancake mix the night before will make a dent in the job come morning.

6. MAKE A DATE WITH YOUR FREEZER

Take the advanced prep one step further by setting aside an hour on a Sunday to prep a couple of freezer-friendly breakfasts. You and your kids will thank yourselves on Monday when you remember that you've stashed a stack of homemade waffles or loaf of zuc-chini bread in the deep freeze.

10 WAYS TO GET YOUR KIDS COOKING BREAKFAST

One surefire method for easing your breakfast burden is to get the kids into the kitchen. Yes, you will pay your dues at first—your countertops will get messy, and you'll have to relinquish some control (kids can be heavy-handed with the sugar spoon)—but in time the payoff is worth the pain. Your kids will gain independence, and you will be off the hook for doing all the work. Here are ten kitchen tasks that, with supervision, even the littlest ones can tackle.

1. Make nut butter toast. Arm kids with a pair of wooden "toaster tongs" and the knowledge that any other tool is unsafe. Nut butter is perfectly spreadable with a dull knife or even the back of a spoon.
2. Scramble a couple of eggs in a pan, with help at first and then independently as they grow older and more competent.
3. Use a butter knife to slice a banana for cereal.
4. Spoon yogurt and granola into a bowl and top with berries.
5. Make a smoothie by measuring ingredients into a blender and letting it run. Teach them not to lift the pitcher off the base until the blade has come to a stop.
6. Use a measuring cup with a handle to scoop breakfast cereal into a bowl.
7. Make muffins together over the weekend, using it as an opportunity to work on math and reading skills.
8. Pitch in with cracking and peeling hard-boiled eggs to have ready in the fridge.
9. Cook a bowl of homemade microwave oatmeal ("Better Than Boxed" Instant Oatmeal, page 77), taking care to use a hot pad or dish towel to transfer the bowl to the table.
10. Stir pancake batter and assist when it comes time to flip pancakes in the pan.

BREAKFAST BATTLES MADE BETTER

Often, prepping and cooking that morning meal is the least of our challenges. Many of us have children with distinct "breakfast personalities" who don't always embrace the meals we've so thoughtfully prepared. Here are a few strategies to help you address the more trying temperaments at your table.

LITTLE MISS "I'M JUST NOT HUNGRY"

This is a tricky one. You want to respect your child's internal hunger meter, but you worry that she needs nourishment before she heads into her day. First, consider whether there are late-night snacking habits that might interfere with her morning appetite or whether the dinner hour has nudged to the later side. Nix after-dinner nibbling and try to move supper a little earlier. Also, ask your child to sit at the breakfast table for at least a few minutes, even if she chooses not to eat. Once she has food in front of her, she may find her appetite after all. Finally, send along a good snack in her backpack, because by mid-morning she may be ready for something more substantial.

LITTLE MISTER PICKY PALATE

You don't want the breakfast table to become a battleground, but dealing with a picky eater at 7 A.M. can be trying. Often, picky kids like to know what to expect, so try a planned meal rotation, being sure to include at least one item you know he'll eat. If, for example, Monday is the day for scrambled eggs, a food he's lukewarm about, serve toast and a glass of milk—two foods he consistently loves—as well. Also, get him involved in the process. Have him pick out a few dishes in this book he'd like to try. Invite him to help bake muffins or blend a smoothie. In my experience, kids are more likely to eat their food if they have a role in preparing it.

LITTLE MISS "I HAVE NO TIME"

This is a common complaint, especially as children get older. Beyond getting kids up ten minutes earlier, you can look for foods that are quick and easy to eat. Do some of the work ahead, such as peeling hard-boiled eggs or cutting up apple slices. In a pinch, pull together meals that can be taken on the road. Egg sandwiches, smoothies packed into to-go cups, and anything wrapped in a tortilla are good places to start.

LITTLE MISTER SNAIL'S-PACE EATER

Being a slow eater is actually a good quality over the long haul, but it can try a parent's patience when it comes to getting a kid to school on time. If you know your child takes a while to eat, get him to the table a little sooner than everyone else so he can go at his own pace. Then, give him a five-minute warning when it's time to think about finishing up.

LITTLE MISS "I ONLY EAT ONE THING"

The downside for "creature of habit" eaters is that by choosing the same meal time and again, they limit the range of nutrients in their diet. That said, it's not the end of the world. It's probably best to chill out a bit first. Second, try to get your child on board with small changes to her current routine, such as adding fruit to her cereal or putting eggs on a tortilla instead of toast. Also, see if you can get her buy-in on a "try it on Tuesday" approach, whereby every Tuesday she agrees to taste something new at breakfast. Who knows? She just may like it.

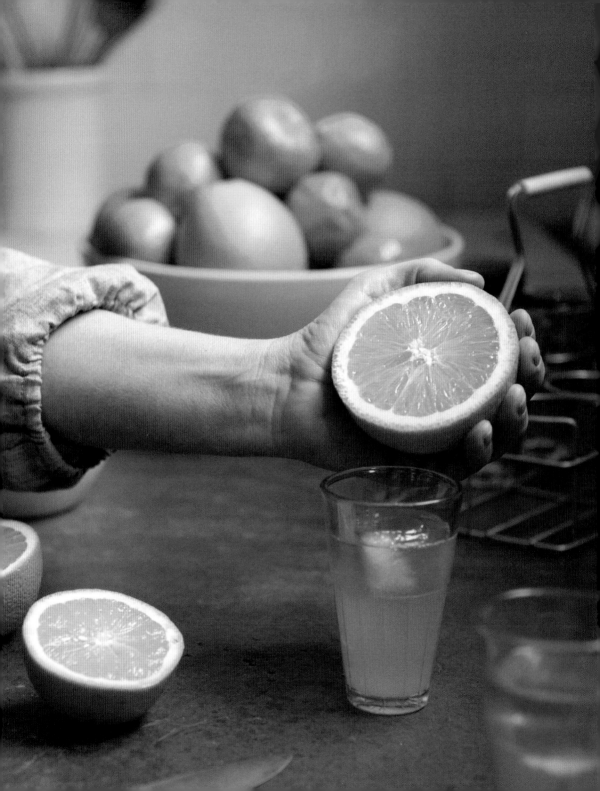

3
SMOOTHIES AND DRINKS

smoothies have been staples in our house since my children were tiny. They're pretty hard to beat for easy meals, considering that all they require are a few ingredients and the ability to push the "on" button of a blender. On mornings when one of the kids declares a breakfast strike, smoothies have often been my secret weapon; the kids can't seem to resist something cold and creamy when it's set right in front of them.

My smoothie-making skills have really evolved over the years. There was a time when I used just a narrow selection of fruit, juice, and ice. Natural ingredients, no doubt, but with clear room for improvement. My repertoire has expanded to include yogurt, milk, tofu, nuts, nut butters, dates, oats, fruit from every season, leafy greens, and other vegetables. Collectively these foods add more nourishment and greater staying power to every glass. The key, of course, is churning out smoothies that taste as delicious as they are nutritious. And these smoothies are just that. My own kids will slurp down every last one in this chapter without crying, "Health food!"

So give them a whirl and, when you do, consider putting your children at the helm of the blender. It's a great place for them to try their hand in the kitchen.

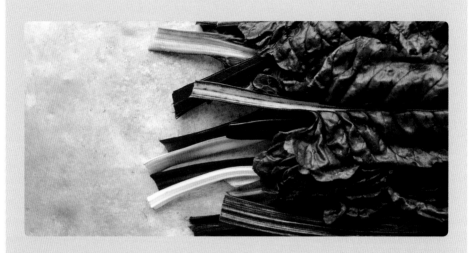

PANTRY STAPLES FOR SMOOTHIE SUCCESS

Smoothies aren't just about fruit juice and ice anymore. On the next page you'll find a chart of ingredients from which to pick and choose depending on the season and your palate. So get busy with your blender. Here's how:

1. Pick a fruit.

2. Add greens or veggies, if desired.

3. Include at least one protein-rich food.

4. Tinker with texture using frozen bananas or other natural thickeners.

5. Add liquid, if needed, to get the blender going.

6. Adjust the sweetness, as needed.

7. Boost the flavor and nutritional value with add-ins and extras.

8. Blend, then pour into glasses.

9. Add toppings, if desired.

10. Drink up!

FRUITS	Pineapple, berries, melon, peaches, apricots, nectarines, pears, apples/applesauce, cherries, oranges/tangerines (seedless), kiwifruits, grapes (seedless), mango, papaya
VEGETABLES	Spinach, kale, cucumber, pumpkin puree, beets, carrots, sweet potatoes
PROTEIN-RICH FOODS	Yogurt; kefir; cottage cheese; milk; soy milk; nut, seed, soy, or peanut butter; nuts or seeds; silken tofu
THICKENERS	Frozen banana; frozen mango; avocado; oats; nut, seed, soy, or peanut butter; ice
LIQUIDS	Coconut water, milk, kefir, carrot juice, vegetable juice, fruit juice, herbal tea, water
SWEETENERS	Dates, prunes, honey, maple syrup
ADD-INS & HEALTHY EXTRAS	Fresh mint, vanilla extract, lime juice, lemon juice, nutmeg, cinnamon, ginger, turmeric, cocoa powder, flaxseed meal, wheat germ, chia seeds, hemp seeds
TOPPINGS	Granola, trail mix, nuts, seeds, dark chocolate shavings, pomegranate seeds, diced fruit

makes 2 servings

STRAWBERRIES AND CREAM SPOON SMOOTHIE

Do me a favor. Don't tell your kids that this smoothie is good for them. "Healthy" is rarely a selling point for anyone, least of all anyone under the age of eighteen. Let them taste it and fall for its creamy texture and scrumptious strawberry flavor rather than the fact that it's full of probiotics or vitamin C. Thicker than a traditional smoothie and crowned with crunchy granola, it's served with a spoon, which makes it more like a meal than a drink. If you prefer a thinner smoothie, add an extra few tablespoons of milk, skip the granola, and slurp it through a straw.

3 TABLESPOONS MILK

¾ CUP PLAIN GREEK YOGURT

¾ CUP FROZEN STRAWBERRIES (FRESH WORK TOO, BUT THE SMOOTHIE WILL BE THINNER)

1 SMALL FROZEN RIPE BANANA, CUT INTO THICK SLICES

1 TABLESPOON PURE MAPLE SYRUP

¼ TEASPOON VANILLA EXTRACT

8 SMALL ICE CUBES

½ CUP GRANOLA

1. Put the milk, yogurt, strawberries, banana, maple syrup, vanilla, and ice into the blender. Run until frothy and smooth. Pour into 2 glasses (you may need to scoop it out with a rubber spatula) and top with the granola. Serve with spoons.

MAKE AHEAD: See "Quick Fix: How to Make and Freeze Smoothies," page 38.

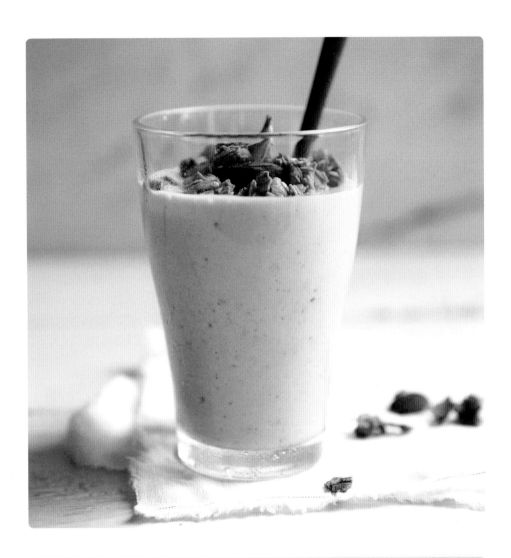

TIP | **A FOOLPROOF FRUIT SMOOTHIE FORMULA**
     | 1 cup yogurt + ½ cup liquid + ¾ cup chopped fruit + 1 frozen ripe banana

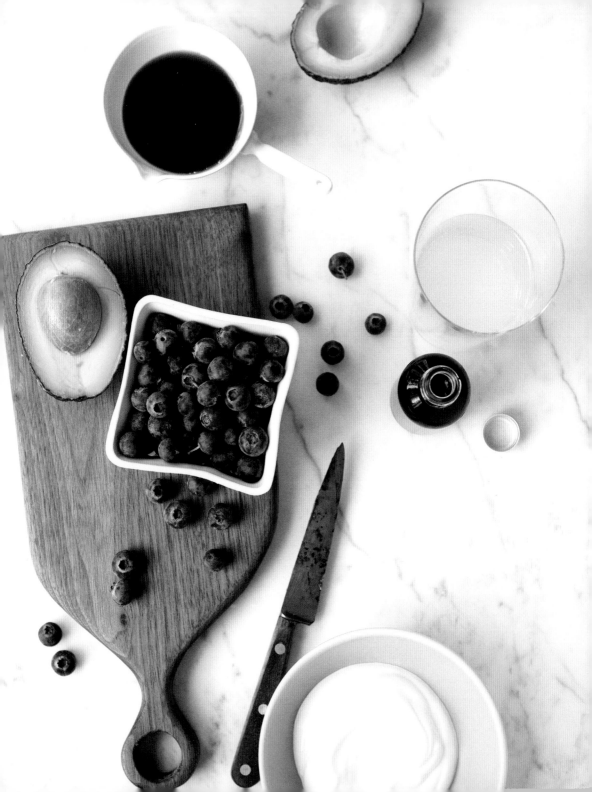

makes 3 servings

BLUEBERRY SUPERFOOD SMOOTHIE

This purple powerhouse is so lip-smackingly tasty, you'd never guess it's packed with superfoods. Blueberries deliver fiber and antioxidants, probiotic-rich kefir lends healthful bacteria, and coconut water is the best natural sports drink I know. Not only that, banana kicks up the potassium, chia seeds add omega-3s, and the avocado? It's full of fiber and good-for-you fats that also give the smoothie the creaminess your kids will never guess came from a plant.

1 CUP PLAIN KEFIR OR PLAIN YOGURT

¾ CUP COCONUT WATER, PLUS MORE IF NEEDED

1 FROZEN RIPE BANANA, CUT INTO THICK SLICES

1 CUP FRESH OR FROZEN BLUEBERRIES

1 SMALL RIPE AVOCADO

½ TEASPOON VANILLA EXTRACT

1 TABLESPOON PLUS 1 TEASPOON PURE MAPLE SYRUP

8 SMALL ICE CUBES

1. Put all the ingredients into a blender and run until creamy and smooth. Add a splash more coconut water to thin the smoothie, if desired. Pour into 3 glasses.

BOOST IT: Top each smoothie with a teaspoon of chia or hemp seeds to add fiber, omega-3 fats, and crunch.

makes 2 or 3 servings

A GREEN SMOOTHIE
(EVEN KIDS WILL LOVE)

Inspiration for this frothy, flavorful drink comes from someone I know only as "The Vitamix Guy." He was at a nutrition conference handing out samples of a green smoothie that was like nothing I'd had before. That is, it didn't taste like someone's backyard lawn. I was smitten and stayed at his booth long enough to gather a rough idea of what was going into that blender. When I got home, I went to work trying to re-create the magic, until I finally nailed it. See for yourself how good a green smoothie can be.

1 MEDIUM SEEDLESS NAVEL ORANGE, PEELED AND SEPARATED INTO 4 SECTIONS

1 CUP CUBED PINEAPPLE, FRESH OR FROZEN AND THAWED

1 PACKED CUP BABY SPINACH

½ FROZEN RIPE BANANA, CUT INTO THICK SLICES

1 TABLESPOON HONEY

10 SMALL ICE CUBES

1. Put all the ingredients into a blender. Blend until creamy, with no obvious pieces of spinach remaining. Pour into 2 or 3 glasses.

   BOOST IT: Add 4 ounces of silken tofu and ½ teaspoon of vanilla extract to the blender to increase the protein and healthful isoflavones.
   ADAPT IT: To minimize the texture, instead of peeling the orange, use a serrated knife to sheer off the entire peel and pith, revealing a bright orange globe of exposed flesh.
   MAKE AHEAD: See "Quick Fix: How to Make and Freeze Smoothies," page 38.

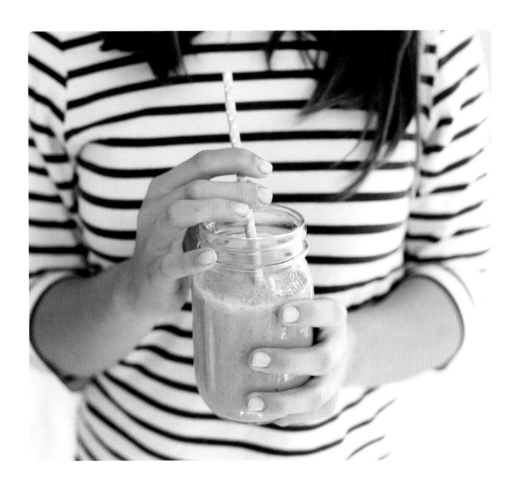

A SMOOTHIE SECRET

I always have a supply of frozen ripe bananas on hand to toss into smoothies because they do wonders for texture. Here's how: allow bananas to get good and ripe, peel them, place in a resealable bag, and store in the freezer. Cut the frozen bananas into thick slices just before adding them to smoothies.

TIP

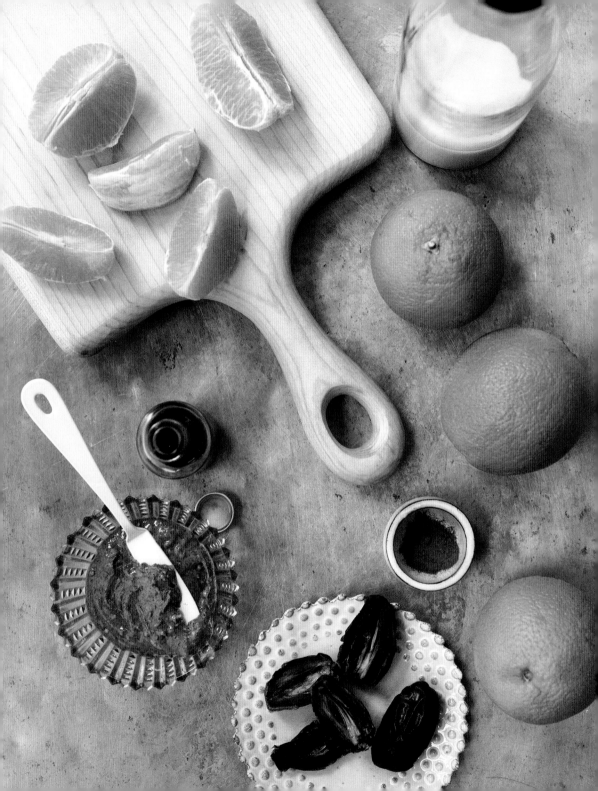

ORANGE ALMOND DATE LASSI

Oranges, almonds, and dates aren't your typical smoothie fixings, but somehow they come together beautifully in this creamy drink that reminds me a little bit of an Orange Julius. I've taken liberties in naming it a lassi because I use milk and almond butter instead of the yogurt that is traditionally used. Like a lassi, the consistency is thinner than a standard smoothie yet plenty luscious and satisfying.

2 LARGE SEEDLESS NAVEL ORANGES, PEELED AND SEPARATED INTO SECTIONS

¾ CUP MILK

3 MEDJOOL DATES, PITTED (SEE "ADAPT IT" BELOW)

2 TABLESPOONS UNSWEETENED ALMOND BUTTER

¼ TEASPOON VANILLA EXTRACT

¼ TEASPOON GROUND CINNAMON

9 SMALL ICE CUBES

1. Be sure to pull off as much white pith as possible from the oranges. Put all the ingredients into a blender and run until smooth, with the dates fully pulverized. Pour into 2 or 3 glasses.

BOOST IT: You can give this a probiotic boost by using kefir instead of milk—just know that the flavor will be more tangy.

ADAPT IT: If your crew doesn't like much texture in their drinks, soften the dates first by soaking them in boiled water for 5 minutes. Lift them out of the water and add them to the blender. Also, instead of peeling the orange, use a serrated knife to sheer off the entire peel and pith, revealing a bright orange globe of exposed flesh.

CITRUS COCONUT WATER COOLER

I'd rather see my kids eating a piece of whole fruit than downing a glass of juice. The sugar and calories in juice are more concentrated, and juice lacks the fiber you get from whole fruit. That said, some mornings call for something cold and sweet and refreshing. This is a tasty OJ alternative that does a bang-up job of hydration. Using juice fresh from an orange means a less processed and better-tasting drink than what you'll find in a carton. The coconut water adds lightness and has about half the calories and half the sugar of standard orange juice. Plus, you'll be meeting more than 50 percent of your daily vitamin C needs.

½ CUP CHILLED COCONUT WATER

1 LARGE NAVEL ORANGE

1. Pour the coconut water into a juice glass. Cut the orange in half and squeeze the juice from both halves into the glass (about ½ cup of juice). Stir.

QUICK FIX | **HOW TO MAKE AND FREEZE SMOOTHIES**
Pour smoothies directly from the blender into a standard ice cube tray. Freeze until solid. Dislodge the cubes from the tray and transfer to a resealable bag. Store in the freezer until ready to use. When the mood for a smoothie strikes, pop out 8 cubes for 1 cup's worth, put them into a glass jar with a lid, and leave on the countertop, covered, for an hour or so. Once thawed, give the jar a vigorous shake to blend the smoothie. You can expedite the process by breaking up the smoothie cubes with a fork after about 30 minutes on the countertop.

makes 1 serving

MILK AND HONEY LATTE

This takes the notion of a comforting mug of warm milk and elevates it to new heights. It's a honey-kissed latte; hold the coffee. The drink is particularly rich and delicious if you indulge in whole milk; however, low-fat and skim milk do froth better. If you're like me and don't happen to own an espresso maker with a milk frother, not to worry. You can make a delightfully warm and bubbly brew on the stove using nothing more than a saucepan and an ordinary whisk.

¾ CUP MILK

1 TEASPOON HONEY

DASH OF GROUND CARDAMOM

1. Pour the milk and honey into a small saucepan and set over medium heat. As the milk warms, swirl the pan a few times to distribute the honey. When the milk feels very warm to the touch, use a small whisk to vigorously beat it for about 30 seconds to create foam. It may help to tilt the pan to the side so the milk pools and is easier to whisk. Once suitably frothy, pour into a mug and top with a dash of cardamom. Serve immediately.

BOOST IT: For the grown-ups in the house, pour the warm milk over ½ cup of hot coffee, and you'll have a Milk and Honey Café au Lait.

ADAPT IT: If cardamom is a new taste for your crew, make this with a dash of cinnamon the first time around, then try it with cardamom once everyone is hooked.

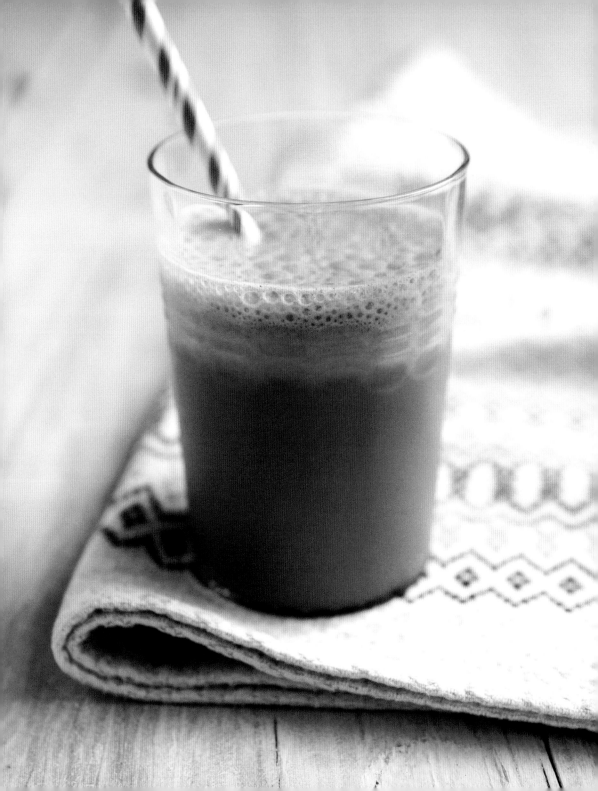

makes 2 or 3 servings

ALMOST INSTANT CHOCOLATE BREAKFAST DRINK

When I first served up this chocolaty drink, my middle daughter, Rosie, loved it so much she drank it before school every morning for two weeks straight. It's a more nourishing and delicious alternative to supermarket powdered breakfast drinks, and it takes only a minute or two to whip up in a blender. Know that it is more a drink than a smoothie, so if you want the signature thickness of a smoothie, add a frozen ripe banana before blending.

1 ½ CUPS MILK

2 TABLESPOONS UNSWEETENED COCOA POWDER

3 TABLESPOONS UNSWEETENED PEANUT BUTTER

1 ½ TABLESPOONS HONEY

7 SMALL ICE CUBES

1. Put all the ingredients into a blender and run until creamy and smooth. Pour into 2 or 3 glasses.

BOOST IT: Add ⅓ cup nonfat dried milk powder before blending. It fortifies the drink with nearly 300 milligrams of calcium and 8 grams of protein, and makes it taste even creamier.

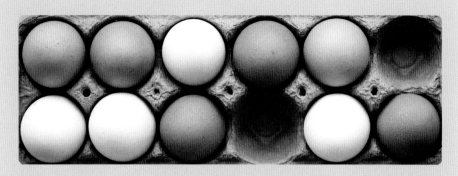

GOOD MORNING LEFTOVERS

Eggs are ideal for using up practically any leftovers you might have on hand. Here are six ideas for making the most of what may already be in your fridge.

COOKED VEGETABLES: A breakfast no-brainer, any cooked vegetables can be chopped up and stirred into scrambled eggs toward the end of cooking, just to warm them through. Or fold veggies inside an omelet along with a favorite cheese.

COOKED GREENS: Leftover steamed or sautéed greens are a tasty base for poached eggs and are excellent inside a breakfast burrito.

COOKED GRAINS: Top leftover polenta, rice, or farro with a simple fried egg, or stir grains into scrambled eggs.

SMOKY MEATS AND FISH: Cured and smoked meats and fish are a particularly good match for eggs. I'm partial to dicing up leftover cooked sausage or ham to throw into a scramble. Smoked salmon or trout are also a treat, particularly rolled into a delicate omelet.

TOFU: Leftover tofu can give a boost of flavor and nutrition to a pan of scrambled eggs.

FRESH HERBS: Chop up basil, chives, cilantro, or other herbs and sprinkle over practically any preparation of eggs, from soft-boiled to shirred, just before serving.

4
EVERYDAY EGGS

"how 'bout an egg?"

This is a common refrain in our house when one of the kids doesn't seem particularly interested in breakfast. I can whip one up in no time, as can they, since scrambled eggs are one of the first foods they learned to cook.

As far as I'm concerned, eggs are one of the world's most perfect foods: housed in a highly portable (albeit delicate) package, nutrient dense, versatile, affordable, and good tasting—what's not to love?

From a nutritional standpoint, an egg is a real gem. Each one has 70 calories, 6 grams of what's considered to be high-quality protein, and a storehouse of other goodies. Unless you have health concerns that dictate otherwise, I suggest you avoid the "egg-white omelet" route and, instead, hang on to every yolk. Sure, it's the egg's source of fat and cholesterol, but it's also home to the majority of the vitamins and minerals. And the fat is important as well, playing a role in the delivery and absorption of key nutrients.

In this chapter, you'll find eggs prepared every which way:

Very simply, such as hard-boiled or baked in a muffin tin
Ahead of time, in mini frittatas or a make-ahead egg pie
Taken to go, in portable pita pockets and egg-topped bagels

Find some old favorites, try a few new ones, and—as my mom would say—"eat your eggs."

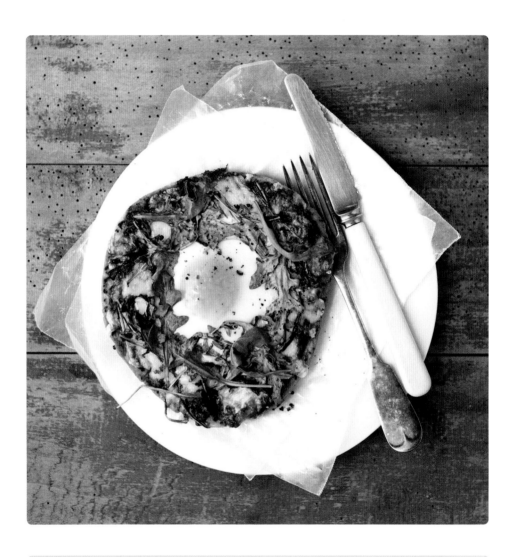

EGG-IN-A-NEST PESTO PIZZA

This little pizza is such a knockout—for both its magazine-cover good looks and its savory flavor—that it's hard to believe it's such a breeze to make. Use pre-grated cheese and prewashed arugula, and you can get this baby bubbling in the oven in a matter of minutes. What results is a crispy pita pizza crust with flavorful toppings, including an oozy egg. It won all three of my kids over at first bite.

ONE 7-INCH WHOLE GRAIN PITA BREAD (DO NOT SPLIT IN HALF)

2 TEASPOONS BASIL PESTO

⅓ CUP COARSELY GRATED MOZZARELLA OR FONTINA CHEESE

½ PACKED CUP BABY ARUGULA

1 LARGE EGG

PINCH OF SALT

1. Move the rack of the oven or toaster oven to the lowest level and preheat to 450°F.
2. Put the pita bread on a baking sheet (small enough to fit in the toaster oven, if using). Spread the pesto evenly over the top of the pita, coming to just shy of the edge. Sprinkle the grated cheese over the pesto. Lay the arugula on top of the cheese to form a ring of greens, leaving a space in the center that's the size of a cooked egg. Crack the egg into the center of the pita so it drops into the space and the ring of arugula holds the egg in place. Sprinkle a pinch of salt over the top.
3. Put the pizza in the oven and bake until the egg is cooked to your liking. For a soft egg, cook until the white is just firm and the yolk is still soft, about 10 minutes. For a firm yolk, cook another 2 minutes or so.
4. Remove from the oven and cut into quarters.

ADAPT IT: Use 2 tablespoons of tomato sauce in place of the pesto.

PERFECT SOFT-COOKED EGGS WITH BUTTERED SOLDIERS

Getting the timing just right for soft eggs, so that the white is cooked and the yolk is still runny, is tricky business. Ever since learning this method from the smart folks at *Cook's Illustrated*, my "on time" results have vastly improved. Really, they're not boiled eggs at all but steamed. The result is a more consistently perfect egg without the tendency for cracked shells, as so often happens when you drop them into boiling water. You can increase the number of eggs as long as you increase the size of the pot, being sure there is a bit of room around each one so they cook evenly. In our house, we serve soft eggs with soldiers, a term the Brits use for buttered toast cut into long strips, which look like tall, thin soldiers, just right for dunking into the center of a tender, golden yolk.

2 COLD EGGS

2 SLICES WHOLE GRAIN SANDWICH BREAD

BUTTER

SALT AND FRESHLY GROUND BLACK PEPPER

1. Fill the bottom of a small saucepan with ½ inch of water. Turn the heat to medium-high and bring the water to a full boil. Quickly (though gently) set the eggs into the pan (using tongs if you prefer). Put on the lid and set a timer for 6½ minutes.

2. While the eggs cook, toast and lightly butter the bread. Cut into ½-inch-wide strips and put on a plate or plates.

3. As soon as the timer rings, put the pan into the sink and run cold water over the eggs for 30 seconds to stop the cooking process.

4. Immediately transfer the eggs to egg

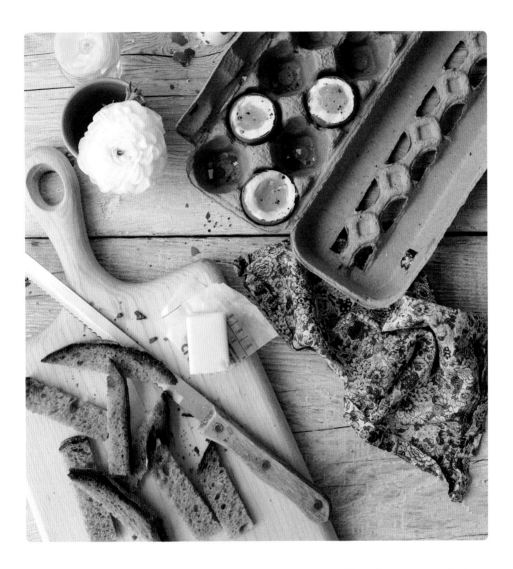

cups, if you have them, or small bowls. Serve with the buttered soldiers and season with salt and pepper, as desired.

ADAPT IT: If you're concerned about serving soft yolks to your little ones, look for eggs pasteurized in the shell.

THE SAFETY OF A SOFT EGG

Growing up, we routinely ate fried and boiled eggs with runny yolks; my parents never thought twice about it. Back then, there was little concern about salmonella, because the incidence of this illness was much lower than it is today. Cooking eggs until the white and yolk are firm is one way to reduce food-borne illness and is something to consider, especially when cooking for very young children. Here are a few other ways to minimize the risk:

- Buy eggs pasteurized in the shell, such as Safest Choice eggs, which are perfectly safe to eat soft or even completely raw.
- Store eggs in the refrigerator, ideally in the center, where it is more consistently cold than on the door.
- Buy eggs from markets that keep them chilled.
- Discard cracked eggs.
- Promptly refrigerate unused or leftover food containing eggs.

makes 3 or 4 servings

GREENS & WHOLE GRAINS SCRAMBLE

With my second and third babies, I had the help of a postpartum doula named Esther, who took such good care of us, it made me want to have a fourth baby just so I could invite her back. Among other skills, she was a terrific cook who made the fluffiest scrambled eggs and fortified them with leftover brown rice. Brilliant. This recipe builds on Esther's eggs with the addition of dark leafy greens. You may think adding sour cream to eggs sounds a bit odd, but try it. You'll be surprised by what just 2 tablespoons can do for flavor.

2 TEASPOONS EXTRA-VIRGIN OLIVE OIL

2 SCALLIONS, THINLY SLICED, WHITE AND LIGHT GREEN PARTS ONLY

1½ PACKED CUPS ROUGHLY CHOPPED SWISS CHARD, KALE, OR COLLARDS WITH TOUGH STEMS REMOVED

6 EGGS, LIGHTLY BEATEN

¼ TO ½ TEASPOON KOSHER SALT

2 TABLESPOONS SOUR CREAM

⅔ CUP COOKED BROWN RICE, FARRO, BARLEY, OR OTHER WHOLE GRAIN OF YOUR CHOICE

1. In a medium skillet, heat the olive oil over medium heat. Add the scallions and sauté until slightly tender, about 1 minute. Add the Swiss chard and continue to sauté until wilted and tender. Add the eggs and ¼ teaspoon salt, and scramble until nearly cooked, with some raw-egg appearance remaining.
2. Remove the pan from heat and gently stir in the sour cream and rice until combined. The heat of the pan will warm the grains and finish cooking the eggs. Add another ¼ teaspoon salt to taste, if desired.

ADAPT IT: Feel free to leave out the grains or greens, and bump up the number of eggs by 1 or 2 if you do.

WEEKDAY HUEVOS

Eggs, beans, and tortillas are three of my most common pantry staples, which means I make some variation of this dish for either breakfast or lunch at least once a week. It's essentially huevos rancheros pared down to the bare bones, yet it is still plenty flavorful. Often, I'll pull out leftover cooked vegetables from the fridge, warm them in a pan, and then tuck them into the tortillas between the beans and fried eggs. Everyone in our house is a fan.

4 CORN TORTILLAS

½ CUP REFRIED BEANS

2 TABLESPOONS MEXICAN SALSA

1 TABLESPOON EXTRA-VIRGIN OLIVE OIL, DIVIDED

4 EGGS

SALT

¼ CUP CRUMBLED COTIJA CHEESE (SEE NOTE)

1. Lay the tortillas on your work surface and spread the beans over them, to the edge. Divide the salsa among the tortillas, spreading it over the beans.

2. Set a large cast iron or nonstick skillet over high heat. Add ½ tablespoon of the olive oil and swirl the pan to coat it evenly. Put the tortillas into the pan. (It's fine if they overlap a little, but if the pan is really crowded, do this in 2 batches.) Cook until the beans are warm to the touch and the tortillas brown a little on the bottom, 2 minutes or so. Transfer the tortillas to serving plates and keep warm near the stove.

3. Reduce the heat to medium-low and add the remaining ½ tablespoon of oil to the pan, swirling to coat. Crack

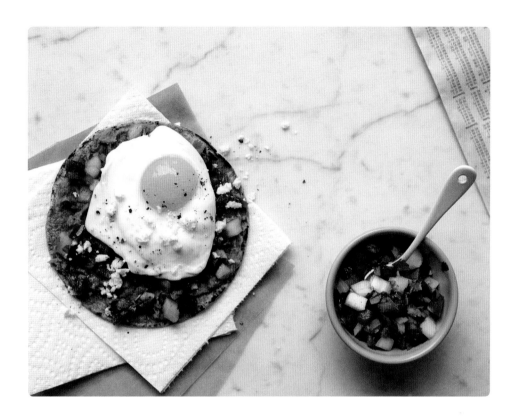

the eggs into the pan, doing your best to keep them from overlapping much. Sprinkle a tiny pinch of salt over the top of each one, and fry to your desired doneness—sunny side up, over easy, over medium, or over hard. Use a spatula to transfer the eggs to the tortillas. Sprinkle the cheese over each one. Serve immediately, as is, with a knife and fork, or fold up like a taco and plan to get messy.

Note: Cotija is a firm, salty Mexican cheese that crumbles. Substitute feta or grated Monterey Jack or Cheddar if you can't find it.

BOOST IT: Add warmed and chopped leftover vegetables to the tortillas before adding the eggs. Alternatively, top each egg with slices of avocado.

makes 3 to 6 servings

MUFFIN TIN BAKED EGGS

Although baked eggs require the forethought to preheat an oven, they're every bit as easy as scrambled or fried. Smearing butter inside the muffin tin and spooning just a teaspoon of milk over the top of the eggs makes all the difference for flavor. They're delicious eaten with a knife and fork, or sandwiched inside an English muffin to take on the road. If you want to get fancy, scatter chopped fresh basil, thyme, or chives in the bottom of the muffin cups before you crack in the eggs. Once cooked, garnish with a touch of the same herb.

1 TABLESPOON BUTTER

6 EGGS

SALT

FRESHLY GROUND BLACK PEPPER

2 TABLESPOONS MILK

1. Preheat the oven to 350°F.
2. Grease 6 muffin cups with the butter.
3. Crack an egg into each of the prepared muffin cups, doing your best not to break the yolks. Add a tiny pinch of salt and a crack of black pepper to the top of each egg. Pour the milk over the eggs, dividing it evenly.
4. Place the muffin tin on the center rack of the oven and bake as follows: For runny yolks, figure 13 to 15 minutes in the oven, until the whites look nearly firm but the yolks are still soft (the eggs will continue to cook after you remove them from the oven). For firm yolks, continue to bake another 2 minutes or so after this point.
5. Remove the pan from the oven and allow to rest on the countertop for 1 minute. Run a knife around the edge of each

egg, gently wedge it out of the pan, and serve as you like.

BOOST IT: Roast a bunch of asparagus while the eggs are cooking. Snap off the tough ends of the stalks, toss with a glug of olive oil and a generous pinch of salt, and spread over a baking sheet. They will take 10 to 15 minutes longer to cook than the eggs, so give them a head start in the oven.

MAKE AHEAD: Cook the eggs until firm and store them in the fridge, where they will keep for a couple of days, then reheat as needed.

QUICK FIX

HAPPINESS IS A HARD-BOILED EGG

To hard-boil eggs, put as many as you like into a pot large enough to accommodate them without crowding. Fill the pot with water so it covers the eggs by 1 inch. Set over high heat and bring to a rolling boil. Cover the pot and remove from heat. Set a timer for 12 minutes. When the timer rings, use a slotted spoon to lift the eggs out of the pot. Serve warm, or transfer to a large bowl of ice water for 1 minute, then store in the refrigerator for up to 1 week.

While it's a breeze to boil up a batch of eggs, slipping off those shells isn't always so easy. Keep in mind that fresh-from-the-market eggs are often the trickiest to peel, so use those for omelets and scrambles, saving eggs that have been in the fridge for a week or more for hard-boiling. To peel, gently tap the large end of the egg on the countertop to crack the shell. There is a little pocket of air at that end, so begin peeling there and work your way down.

makes 3 servings

ONE-EYED JACK IN A BAGEL

One-Eyed Jack, Winkie, Eggy Bread, Egg-in-a-Hole, Bull's-Eye—whatever you call an egg cracked into the center of a slice of bread and cooked, it's a truly efficient meal for filling a hungry belly, and it certainly demands little of the cook. This recipe puts a twist on the original by subbing an all-time-favorite kid food for the toast: a bagel. The key is to slice it into three rounds instead of two, which allows for a crispy outside and a more even balance of egg to bread. Cook this long enough for the yolk to go firm and it can be a breakfast-to-go.

1 BAGEL (NOT PRE-SLICED), PREFERABLY WHOLE GRAIN

1 TABLESPOON BUTTER

3 EGGS

SALT

FRESHLY GROUND BLACK PEPPER

1. Use a serrated knife to cut the bagel into 3 rounds. Put the bagel slices on a cutting board. Use a round cookie cutter that is about 1½ inches in diameter to cut a bigger hole (around the existing one) in the center of each bagel. You can make the bigger hole using a knife if you don't have a cookie cutter.

2. Set a large skillet over medium-high heat and melt the butter, tilting the pan so it coats the bottom. Put the bagel slices in the pan, cut-side down.

3. Crack an egg into the center of each bagel slice, allowing it to settle inside the hole. Sprinkle a small pinch of salt and a crack of black pepper over the top of each egg. Drop the heat down to medium and cook the eggs until the bagel browns lightly on the bottom and

the egg whites begin to set, about 3 minutes. Use a spatula to flip the bagels over. Season with salt and black pepper on the second side and continue to cook until the yolks are done to your liking.

4. Use a spatula to transfer the egg-filled bagels to serving plates. Serve with a knife and fork.

BOOST IT: Top with a couple of slices of ripe tomato or avocado and a tiny pinch of salt.

CUTTING BAGELS DOWN TO SIZE

Bagels are far bigger today than they were a generation ago. To keep portion sizes in check, I like to cut bagels into three rounds instead of two. That way, you can have a top and a bottom with room in between for nourishing fillings. Save the middle slice for breakfast toast or for making a One-Eyed Jack in a Bagel.

VEGGIE SCRAMBLE PITA POCKETS

Scrambled eggs are the perfect vehicle for recycling last night's supper. Here, I've worked leftover vegetables into egg pockets that just need a crumble of feta cheese to bring it all together. Any vegetables will do, really, be it sautéed zucchini, roasted sweet potatoes, or steamed broccoli. Just be sure to chop it up small so it's easy to tuck inside the pita.

2 TEASPOONS EXTRA-VIRGIN OLIVE OIL

5 EGGS, LIGHTLY BEATEN

¼ TEASPOON KOSHER SALT

FRESHLY GROUND BLACK PEPPER

1 CUP DICED LEFTOVER COOKED VEGETABLES

⅓ CUP CRUMBLED FETA CHEESE

TWO 7-INCH WHOLE GRAIN PITA BREADS

1. Set a medium skillet over medium heat. Add the olive oil and tilt the pan to coat the bottom. Add the eggs, salt, and a few cracks of pepper. Gently scramble the eggs until nearly cooked. Add the vegetables, stir, and remove from the heat. Sprinkle the feta over the eggs.

2. Heat the pita breads in a toaster just long enough to warm them (you don't want them crispy). Cut the pitas in half and fill each half with the egg mixture.

BOOST IT: If you have fresh basil, parsley, or chives on hand, chop up 1 to 2 tablespoons and add it along with the vegetables.

ADAPT IT: You can cut back on the amount of vegetables or leave them out altogether. If you do, be sure to add a couple more eggs to the scramble so you'll have enough filling for the pitas. Feel free to substitute any favorite grated cheese for the feta.

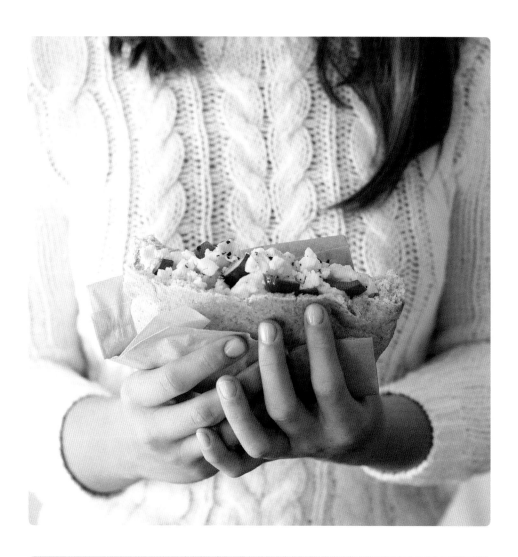

TIP | Store uncooked eggs in the fridge and use them within five weeks of the "sell by" date on the carton.

makes 6 frittatas; 3 to 6 servings

MAKE-AHEAD MINI SPINACH FRITTATAS

If anyone is wondering about the vibrant yellow of these frittatas, you can tell them it's not the result of neon yolks from bionic eggs. It's from the turmeric, a mildly fragrant spice that adds a golden hue and amazing flavor, and that shows real promise as a natural anti-inflammatory. This recipe draws inspiration from a Persian egg dish called *kookoo* (or *kuku*) that's traditionally made with loads of bright green herbs and turmeric. My version calls for spinach instead—specifically, frozen chopped spinach, to minimize prep time. Make these a day ahead, and wake up to a mega-satisfying breakfast that you can tuck into a lunch box, too.

6 EGGS

¼ CUP MILK

5 OUNCES FROZEN CHOPPED SPINACH, DEFROSTED

2 SCALLIONS, THINLY SLICED, WHITE AND LIGHT GREEN PARTS ONLY

1 ¼ TEASPOONS GROUND TURMERIC

½ TEASPOON KOSHER SALT

½ CUP CRUMBLED FETA CHEESE

1. Preheat the oven to 325°F. Line 6 muffin cups with cupcake liners and generously grease the liners with oil or nonstick cooking spray.

2. Crack the eggs into a medium bowl. Add the milk and whisk until combined. Drain the defrosted spinach well, pressing out as much of the liquid as you can. Add the spinach, scallions, turmeric, and salt to the eggs and whisk together. Add the feta and stir gently until just combined.

3. Divide the egg mixture among the 6 muffin cups, filling them nearly to the

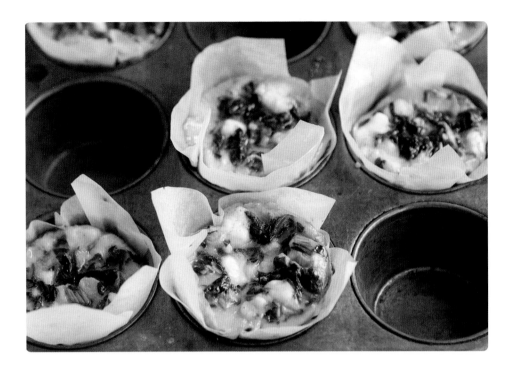

top. I use a measuring cup with a handle for this.

4. Bake the frittatas for about 30 minutes, until just firm at the top, with no raw egg appearance.

5. Remove the muffin tin from the oven. Cool for a few minutes, then run a knife around the edges to wedge the frittatas from the muffin tin. Serve warm, or allow the frittatas to come to room temperature before covering and storing in the refrigerator.

BOOST IT: Swap out the spinach for 1 cup of any favorite cooked, diced vegetables, such as zucchini, bell peppers, or mushrooms.

MAKE AHEAD: This recipe can be doubled easily. Keep leftovers in the fridge for up to 3 days, or wrap them in plastic, put them in a resealable bag, and store them in the freezer.

PIMENTO AND CHEDDAR EGG PIE

My friend Mary Ellen gave me this recipe, at least a version of it, that she inherited from her mother, who got it from a neighbor, who got it from who knows where. It's just that sort of recipe: one worth sharing. While Mary Ellen always makes it for company, I've found that it's just right for a weekday breakfast because it's a one-bowl affair that can be made ahead. The result is a cheesy, pimento-flecked egg dish reminiscent of a frittata.

6 EGGS

1 CUP SMALL-CURD COTTAGE CHEESE

¼ CUP MILK

2 TABLESPOONS BUTTER, MELTED

¼ CUP WHOLE WHEAT OR ALL-PURPOSE FLOUR, SPOONED AND LEVELED

1 TEASPOON BAKING POWDER

¾ TEASPOON KOSHER SALT

ONE 4-OUNCE JAR DICED PIMENTOS, DRAINED (SEE NOTE)

⅔ CUP (PACKED) COARSELY GRATED SHARP CHEDDAR CHEESE

1. Preheat the oven to 350°F. Grease an 8 × 8-inch pan with oil or nonstick cooking spray.
2. Crack the eggs into a medium bowl and whisk well. Add the cottage cheese, milk, butter, flour, baking powder, and salt. Whisk again to combine. Add the pimentos and cheese, and stir to combine. Pour the egg mixture into the prepared pan and bake 30 to 35 minutes, until the egg is just firm to the touch at the center. Remove from the oven and allow to cool for at least 5 minutes. Cut into squares and serve.

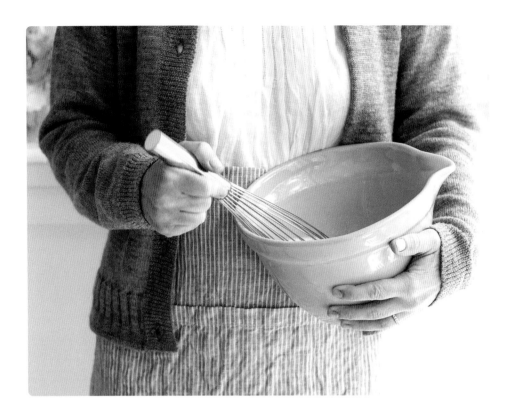

Note: Pimentos are mild red chiles available in small jars in the supermarket where the olives, capers, and roasted red peppers are sold.

BOOST IT : Add 1 cup of cooked broccoli (in 1- to 1½-inch florets) to the egg mixture after the pimentos and cheese. Stir again and pour into the prepared pan.

ADAPT IT: If your kids aren't keen on pimentos, leave them out.

MAKE AHEAD: Instead of cooking this right away, cover the bowl with plastic wrap and store it in the fridge overnight. In the morning, stir the mixture again, pour into a greased pan, and bake as instructed. Once cooked, the egg pie will keep in the fridge for up to 3 days. Serve cold or reheat.

makes 1 serving

SWEET EGG CREPE WITH
CHERRY JAM AND CRÈME FRAÎCHE

I wasn't sure what to call this delicate egg dish that lands somewhere between an omelet and a crepe, with a tiny dash of soufflé in there somewhere. One thing I am sure about is that it is no ordinary egg dish. When you want to give someone the royal treatment one morning, this is the call. It's not as straightforward as a standard omelet because it requires extra elbow grease to whip the egg whites and a deft hand to flip it over. Don't worry if you don't get it right the first time. It will still be tasty, even if it's not perfectly pretty.

1 EGG

1 TABLESPOON MILK

1 TEASPOON SUGAR

¼ TEASPOON VANILLA EXTRACT

1 TABLESPOON BUTTER

1 TABLESPOON CHERRY JAM OR OTHER TANGY JAM OF YOUR CHOICE

1 TABLESPOON CRÈME FRAÎCHE

1. Separate the egg, dropping the white into a supremely clean, medium metal bowl and the yolk into a separate medium bowl.

2. Add the milk, sugar, and vanilla to the bowl with the yolk, whisk until combined, and set aside.

3. Using a clean wire whisk, beat the egg white vigorously by hand until it turns thick and frothy (halfway between unwhipped and soft peaks) and nearly white in color, 1 to 2 minutes.

4. Add the whipped white to the yolk mixture and gently fold together.

5. Set a 9- or 10-inch nonstick or cast iron skillet over medium heat. Add

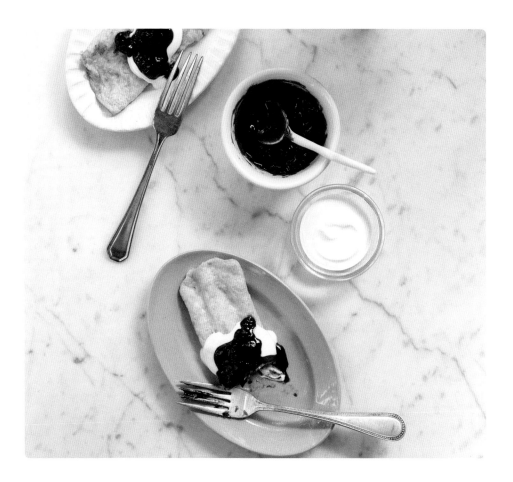

the butter and melt, swirling to coat the pan. Pour in the egg mixture, tilting the pan so it runs to the edges and spreads out evenly. You may need to use a spoon to help it a bit. Cook until the egg is just barely golden, set, and sturdy enough to flip. Wedge a large spatula underneath the egg and turn it over. Cook on the second side until barely golden and cooked through. With the aid of the spatula, roll the egg so it folds over twice, then tilt the pan and allow it to roll onto a plate.

6. Top with cherry jam and crème fraîche.

TOP TEN ADD-INS TO MAKE COLD CEREAL COUNT

Ready-to-eat cereal is part of the breakfast rotation for most households these days. Make more of every bowl by raiding your pantry for creative toppings. Here are ten ideas for adding texture, flavor, and nutrients. They're dynamite on hot cereal too.

1. Blueberries, raspberries, or blackberries—Fiber and antioxidant rich, these petite fruits require no slicing or dicing. Just wash a handful to top off your favorite flakes.

2. Slivered or sliced almonds—These add appealing crunch along with calcium, fiber, and vitamin E.

3. Flaxseed meal—To derive all the nutrients from flaxseeds, it's best to eat them ground. Sprinkle a tablespoon over a bowl of cereal to add a dose of healthy omega-3 fats.

4. Pepitas (shelled pumpkin seeds) or sunflower seeds—These add texture, fiber, and healthy fats to keep you filled up longer.

5. Chopped walnuts—Nutrient packed, walnuts will up your antioxidants and omega-3s.

6. Sliced banana—A cereal-topping classic, this tropical fruit is prized for its natural sweetness and reputation as a potassium powerhouse.

7. Wheat germ—Add a tablespoon or two to your breakfast bowl for more fiber, protein, and a host of other nutrients.

8. Trail mix—The combination of nuts, seeds, and dried fruits means additional fiber, healthy fats, and plenty of staying power. Look for one without added sugar.

9. Sliced peaches or nectarines—In season, a ripe peach or nectarine adds sweetness, vitamin C, and a burst of color.

10. Chia or hemp seeds—These seeds are protein dense and fiber rich, and they supply coveted omega-3 fats. A little goes a long way, so even just a tablespoon will do.

5

GRANOLA, OATS, AND BREAKFAST GRAINS

growing up, we often began mornings with bowls of creamy oatmeal or warm farina cereal. My mom would brew up a generous pot and leave it on the stove with brown sugar and raisins to sprinkle over the top. To this day, when I think of hot cereal, I think of home.

With my own kids, I've continued the tradition, expanding our repertoire into new territory. We've tinkered with millet and teff, made breakfast rice pudding in the slow cooker, and eaten oats in every imaginable fashion.

Of course, it's not just my family who leans on grains for breakfast. So do cultures the world over, and for good reason: these are some of the most affordable and convenient foods money can buy. Whole grain cereal is supremely nourishing and enormously satisfying, not to mention just plain delicious.

The recipes here include a few old favorites, such as my time-tested granola and an oatmeal recipe that a third grader could tackle. Once you've got those under your belt, stretch a little. Try steel-cut oats with savory toppings instead of sweet, consider quinoa as suitable for breakfast as it is for supper, or after all these years of eating granola, give muesli a go.

MY GIRLS' GRANOLA

I've been making this granola since I was in my twenties when, as an enthusiastic new bride, I gave it out as Christmas gifts. Over time, the recipe has evolved, becoming as much a staple in our home as any other food in the pantry. If you've never made granola before, you may be surprised by how easy it is. A few batches in and you'll be hooked, in part because coconut granola browning in your oven will make the whole kitchen smell like a bakery. When it's cooling on the countertop, I can't keep my girls from snatching handfuls off of the baking sheets.

3½ CUPS OLD-FASHIONED ROLLED OATS (NOT QUICK OATS)

1 CUP CHOPPED WALNUTS

¾ CUP UNSWEETENED SHREDDED COCONUT

¾ TEASPOON GROUND CARDAMOM

½ TEASPOON KOSHER SALT

½ CUP PLUS 1 TABLESPOON PURE MAPLE SYRUP

¼ CUP EXTRA-VIRGIN OLIVE OIL

2 TABLESPOONS BUTTER, MELTED

1 CUP DRIED CRANBERRIES

1. Preheat the oven to 300°F. Line a large baking sheet with parchment paper or a silicone baking mat.

2. In a large bowl, stir together the oats, walnuts, coconut, cardamom, and salt.

3. In a medium bowl, whisk together the maple syrup, olive oil, and melted butter.

4. Pour the maple syrup mixture over the oats mixture and stir with a spoon or mix with your hands until combined.

5. Distribute the mixture evenly over the baking sheet. Bake about 50 minutes, until deeply golden brown, rotating the baking sheet a half-turn halfway

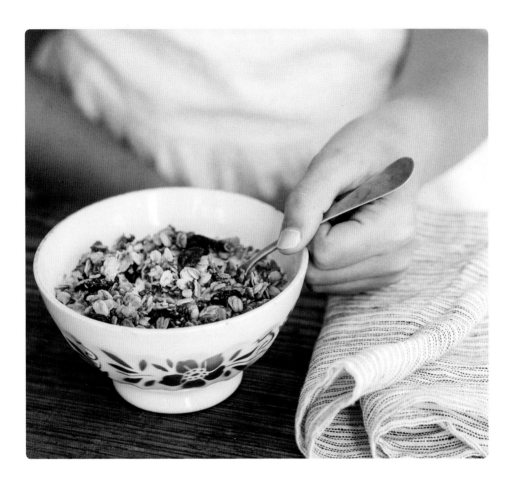

through. Feel free to stir after 25 minutes if it looks like the granola is not browning evenly. Remove from the oven and allow to cool completely on the baking sheet. Scatter the cranberries over the top and transfer the granola to an airtight container.

ADAPT IT: Feel free to substitute another favorite nut and dried fruit for the walnuts and cranberries.

MAKE AHEAD: Granola will keep well for several weeks at room temperature or for several months in the freezer in a resealable bag with the air pressed out.

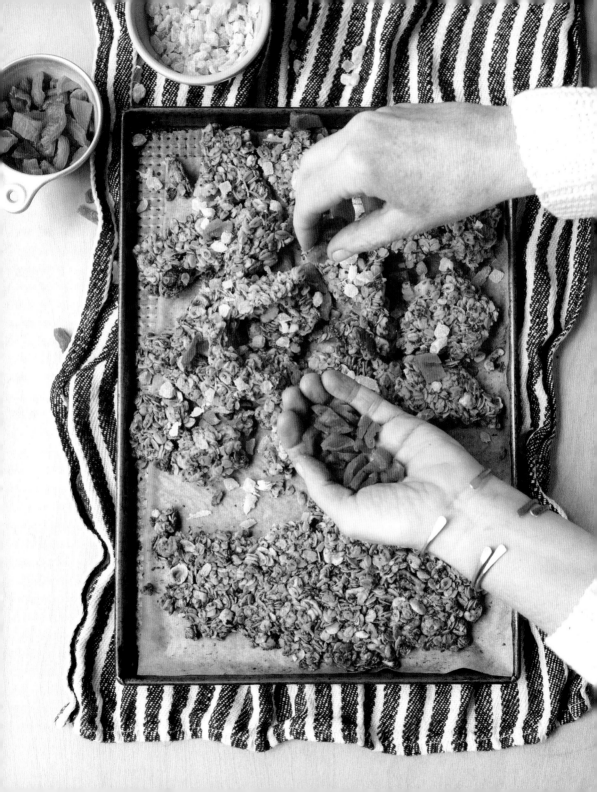

APRICOT GINGER CLUSTER GRANOLA

Scan the list of ingredients in this recipe—honey, flaxseed, spelt, and hemp—and you may worry that it's a little too "hippie" for you. However, the taste is anything but. All the wholesome goodies bake up like a giant granola bar that you break into crunchy clusters. Tossing in dried apricots and crystallized ginger adds a sweet/spicy flavor and pleasing chew. Consider it granola "finger food," which means it's as good on the go as it is in a cereal bowl under a pool of cold milk.

2 CUPS OLD-FASHIONED ROLLED OATS (NOT QUICK OATS)

1 ½ CUPS SPELT, QUINOA, BARLEY, OR RYE FLAKES (SEE NOTE)

⅓ CUP OAT FLOUR OR WHOLE WHEAT FLOUR, SPOONED AND LEVELED

½ CUP FLAXSEED MEAL, WHEAT BRAN, OR WHEAT GERM

¼ CUP HEMP, SESAME, OR CHIA SEEDS

1 ½ CUPS ROUGHLY CHOPPED NUTS, SUCH AS PECANS, ALMONDS, WALNUTS, AND/OR HAZELNUTS

¼ CUP FINELY CHOPPED CRYSTALLIZED GINGER

¾ TEASPOON KOSHER SALT

⅓ CUP HONEY

⅓ CUP PURE MAPLE SYRUP

½ CUP EXTRA-VIRGIN OLIVE OIL

2 TEASPOONS VANILLA EXTRACT

1 EGG

1 CUP ROUGHLY CHOPPED DRIED APRICOTS

1. Preheat the oven to 300°F. Line a large baking sheet with parchment paper or a silicone baking mat.

2. In a large bowl, stir together the rolled

oats, spelt flakes, oat flour, flaxseed meal, hemp seeds, nuts, crystallized ginger, and salt.

3. In a medium bowl, whisk together the honey, maple syrup, olive oil, and vanilla. Pour the syrup mixture over the oats and stir well to thoroughly coat. Crack the egg over the granola and thoroughly mix it into the oats, being sure the white and yolk are evenly incorporated. Your hands can be useful for this.

4. Distribute the mixture evenly over the baking sheet. Use your hands to press the granola down firmly in the pan so it looks like a large granola bar that covers the majority of the baking sheet. Bake about 40 minutes, until deeply golden brown, rotating the baking sheet a half-turn halfway through.

5. Remove from the oven and allow to cool completely on the baking sheet. Once cool, break the granola into many 2- to 3-bite chunks. Scatter the dried apricots over the granola and transfer to an airtight container. Store in the fridge, where it will stay extra crunchy.

Note: These grain flakes look just like rolled oats and can be found in the bulk bin or breakfast cereal section of some health food and specialty stores. If you can't find them, feel free to use old-fashioned rolled oats instead.

MAKE AHEAD: This granola will keep for several weeks in the fridge. It stores well for several months in the freezer in a resealable bag with the air pressed out.

LOVE YOUR GRANOLA . . . JUST NOT TOO MUCH

Nobody is crazier for granola than the folks living under my roof, which is why I do my best to keep a jar stocked in the pantry. But here's the rub: wholesome though it may be, the nuts, seeds, dried fruits, and oil mean granola can pack a lot of calories into a relatively small portion. For most people, keeping the serving to ½ cup or less will suffice, providing ample nutrition to fuel a morning, particularly when paired with milk or yogurt and fresh fruit.

makes about 6 cups

DARK CHOCOLATE RASPBERRY MUESLI

As much as I always wanted to love muesli—a mixture of oats, nuts, and dried fruits that hails from the Swiss Alps—I could never quite get there. Raw grains soaked in milk? It just didn't do it for me. That was until I tried a version at a small hotel in Budapest during a family vacation one summer. The oats, nuts, and seeds were all lightly toasted, giving it appealing crunch. And the kicker? The muesli was dotted with bittersweet chocolate, just enough to hold my interest. Sold! I've been making my own ever since. If you're not a muesli lover yet, this recipe may just make you a convert.

2½ CUPS OLD-FASHIONED ROLLED OATS (NOT QUICK OATS)

½ CUP SLIVERED ALMONDS OR CHOPPED NUTS OF YOUR CHOICE

⅓ CUP RAW PEPITAS (SHELLED PUMPKIN SEEDS)

1 CUP WHOLE GRAIN CEREAL FLAKES, SUCH AS UNCLE SAM CEREAL, OR CRISPY BROWN RICE CEREAL

¾ CUP FREEZE-DRIED RASPBERRIES OR STRAWBERRIES (SEE NOTE)

½ CUP FINELY CHOPPED BITTERSWEET CHOCOLATE (ABOUT 2 OUNCES)

¼ CUP CHIA OR HEMP SEEDS

1. Preheat the oven to 350°F.

2. Combine the oats, almonds, and pepitas on a baking sheet and spread out. Bake for about 12 minutes, until the oats are lightly toasted and the pepitas begin to brown. Remove from the oven and allow to cool for 15 minutes.

3. Transfer the oats, almonds, and pepitas to a large bowl. Add the cereal, freeze-dried raspberries, chocolate, and chia seeds. Stir well. The chocolate may melt slightly and form little clumps, which is part of the muesli's appeal.

4. Store in an airtight container. Shake the container to evenly distribute the ingredients before serving with milk or yogurt.

Note: If you can't find freeze-dried berries, use dried cherries, dried cranberries, or raisins.

BOOST IT: Top muesli with sliced banana, fresh berries, or another favorite fruit.

ADAPT IT: Mix ¼ cup muesli into your child's favorite breakfast cereal to introduce the new flavors. Over time, he or she may develop a taste for it straight up.

MAKE AHEAD: Muesli will keep for up to 2 weeks at room temperature.

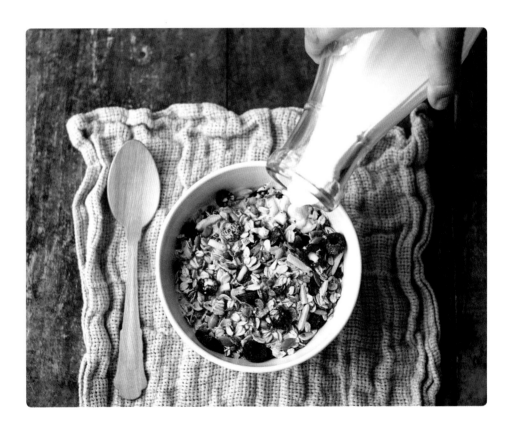

GOOD MORNING TRAIL MIX

OK, so muesli may sound a little too foreign and granola may sound too hippie, but *trail mix*? That's a term any child who has ever been on a day hike or a camping trip can relate to. Keep a jar of this no-fuss mix on hand for days when the kids are bounding for the bus and the grown-ups are racing to a meeting. It's easily adaptable, so tailor it to suit your palate and your pantry, making it your very own.

⅔ CUP NON-FLAKE CEREAL, SUCH AS BARBARA'S PUFFINS
OR MULTIGRAIN SPOONFULS OR A CHEX-TYPE CEREAL

⅔ CUP GRANOLA

⅓ CUP HAZELNUTS, ALMONDS, PEANUTS, OR CASHEWS

⅓ CUP WALNUTS OR PECANS

⅓ CUP ROASTED SUNFLOWER SEEDS OR PEPITAS (SHELLED PUMPKIN SEEDS), SALTED OR UNSALTED

½ CUP FREEZE-DRIED FRUIT, SUCH AS APPLE, RASPBERRIES, MANGO, OR PINEAPPLE

⅓ CUP DRIED FRUIT, SUCH AS RAISINS, CRANBERRIES, OR CHERRIES

1. Combine all the ingredients in a large bowl using your hands or a spoon. Transfer to an airtight container or resealable bag.

BOOST IT: Down a glass of milk with the trail mix for added protein, calcium, and hydration.

ADAPT IT: To sweeten the deal, add ¼ cup bittersweet chocolate chips.

MAKE AHEAD: Portion out ½ cup servings into wax-paper snack bags or reusable containers for easy, grab-and-go breakfasts.

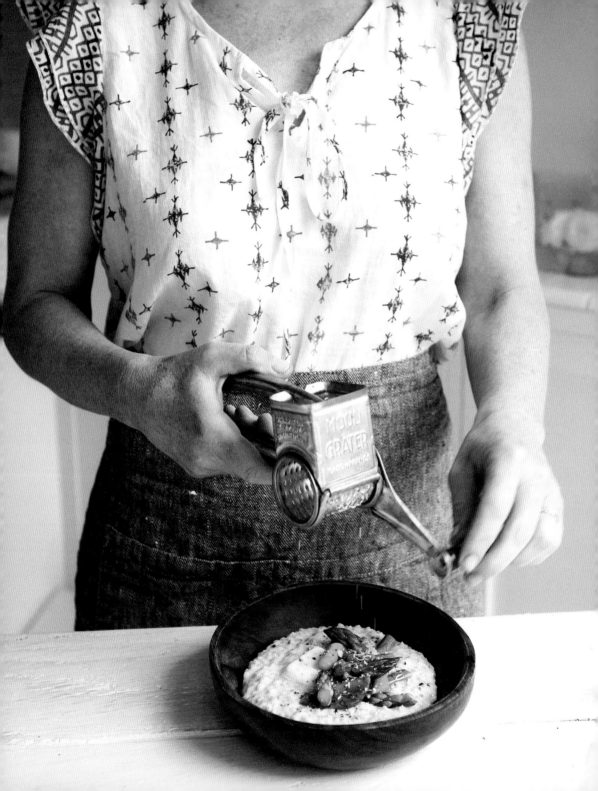

SAVORY OVERNIGHT OATS

In the world of oats, the steel-cut variety, also known as "Irish oats," is at the top of the "good-for-you" food chain. I'm crazy about them, but I'm not so fond of the fact that they take *forever* to cook. It's the risotto of breakfast foods. And who has time for risotto at the crack of dawn? This overnight method cuts morning cooking time down dramatically and results in warm and creamy oats that will fuel you until lunchtime. Here, I do them up savory instead of sweet, with butter, salt, and black pepper instead of brown sugar or raisins. If you've never tried oats this way, do.

2¼ CUPS WATER

1 CUP MILK

1 CUP STEEL-CUT OATS

½ TEASPOON KOSHER SALT

1 OR 1⅓ TABLESPOONS BUTTER

FRESHLY GROUND BLACK PEPPER

FLAKY SALT, SUCH AS MALDON OR FLEUR DE SEL (OPTIONAL)

1. The night before, pour the water and milk into a medium saucepan. Set over medium-high heat and bring it just barely to a boil. Watch the pot closely because it can quickly bubble over. Add the oats and salt, stir, and lower the heat. Gently simmer for 1 minute, stirring a few times. Remove from the heat, cover with a lid, and place in the refrigerator to chill overnight.

2. In the morning, return the pot to the stove over high heat. As soon as the oat mixture comes to a boil, lower the heat. Gently simmer, stirring occasionally, until the liquid is mostly absorbed and the oats are still a little chewy, 8 to 10

minutes. It may look rather soupy, but it will thicken as it cools.

3. Divide into serving bowls and top each one with a dab of butter and a few cracks of black pepper. Add a small pinch of flaky salt to each bowl, if desired.

BOOST IT: Top each bowl of oats with a fried egg just before serving. Alternatively (or in addition), add leftover warmed vegetables and shaved Parmesan. Sautéed mushrooms and leafy greens are particularly tasty.

ADAPT IT: If eating oats the savory way is too much of a stretch, no problem. Enjoy this how you normally might, with maple syrup or brown sugar. You may want to scale back the amount of salt to ¼ teaspoon.

DOUBLE UP

Leftover oatmeal and other hot cereal keep well for several days in the fridge, so make a double batch. Simply reheat on the stove or in the microwave, adding milk or water as needed. Alternatively, chilled oatmeal, polenta, or grits can be cut into thick slabs and browned in an oil-slicked skillet. Top with a pinch of salt and a drizzle of olive oil or maple syrup. Delicious.

"BETTER THAN BOXED" INSTANT OATMEAL

This recipe is a more economical, eco-friendly, and healthier alternative to most store-bought packets of microwave oatmeal. Simply make up a generous jar, keep a one-third-cup measure nearby, and then you (or your kids) can scoop up a serving whenever the mood for a simple, warm breakfast strikes. Be sure to shake the mix before using, and cook the oatmeal in a deep cereal bowl because it can bubble up and overflow when heated.

OATMEAL MIX

2 CUPS OLD-FASHIONED ROLLED OATS (NOT QUICK OATS)

½ CUP DRIED FRUIT, SUCH AS RAISINS, DRIED CRANBERRIES, DICED DRIED APPLES, OR DICED DRIED APRICOTS

½ CUP SLIVERED OR CHOPPED ROASTED NUTS

½ TEASPOON GROUND CINNAMON

TO MAKE ONE SERVING

ROUNDED ⅓ CUP OATMEAL MIX

⅔ CUP WATER

MILK AND/OR PURE MAPLE SYRUP, FOR SERVING

1. To make the oatmeal mix, put the oats, dried fruit, nuts, and cinnamon into a large jar or resealable bag with a bit of extra room. Shake well until all the ingredients are thoroughly combined.

2. To prepare one serving of oatmeal, scoop ⅓ cup of the Oatmeal Mix into a deep, microwave-safe cereal bowl. (If the bowl is too shallow, the oatmeal may overflow when it cooks.) Add ⅔

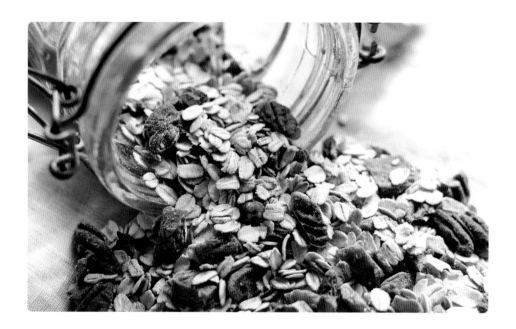

cup water and stir well. Place the bowl in the microwave and cook on high for about 2 minutes, until the water is absorbed and the oats are tender. Remove the bowl from the microwave and stir. The oatmeal will thicken as it cools. If you prefer thicker oatmeal, scale back the water by 1 or 2 tablespoons. Add milk and/or maple syrup, if desired.

BOOST IT: For a creamier cereal that's higher in protein and calcium, cook the oats with milk instead of water as follows: The night before, stir together a rounded ⅓ cup of the Oatmeal Mix with ⅔ cup milk in a microwave-safe cereal bowl. Cover with plastic wrap and store in the refrigerator overnight. In the morning, remove the plastic and microwave on high for about 2 minutes.

MAKE AHEAD: Instead of storing all the mix in a single jar, make individual oatmeal packets by filling each of 8 wax-paper bags with a rounded ⅓ cup of the Oatmeal Mix, making it even easier for kids to prep a bowl in the morning.

QUICK FIX

BREAKFAST CEREAL: THE BEST OF THE BUNCH

As much as I might like to start every morning with a homemade breakfast, some days boxed cereal is as good as it gets. Unfortunately, the cereal aisle leaves much to be desired from a nutrition standpoint, so be thoughtful about what you buy. Look for brands with a whole grain listed as the first ingredient, such as whole wheat, brown rice, or oats. Also, keep an eye on calories, because some cereals pack a lot of them into a small portion. Last, aim for at least 3 grams of fiber and 5 or fewer grams of sugar per serving. Here are nine cereals that fill the bill:

UNCLE SAM ORIGINAL CEREAL: This is a winner for its fiber content, with 10 grams per serving. The fact that it has just four ingredients is also a plus.

NATURE'S PATH FLAX PLUS: A good one if you're looking for a flake cereal, because it keeps the sugar down and the fiber up, at 4 grams and 5 grams, respectively.

BARBARA'S ORIGINAL PUFFINS: A kid favorite that tastes like a "sugar" cereal even with just 5 grams per serving.

BARBARA'S MULTIGRAIN SPOONFULS: Another one with plenty of kid appeal that's made with oat and corn flour.

"O" CEREALS, SUCH AS CHEERIOS: The kid classic with a mere 1 gram of sugar per serving.

ORIGINAL KIX: Made with whole grain corn, this is another popular choice for little ones, and boasts just 3 grams of sugar.

POST GRAPE-NUTS: This tiny cereal has an impressive 7 grams of fiber and 6 grams of protein per serving, but keep an eye on the portion, because it's 210 calories per half cup.

WEETABIX: This UK brand with a crunchy texture has made its way over the pond and has only 2 grams of sugar per serving.

TRADER JOE'S SHREDDED BITE SIZE WHEATS: This has just two little ingredients and no sugar at all. Even if you add a teaspoon of sugar to your own bowl, it will still come in under that 5 gram goal.

HAM AND CHEESE BREAKFAST POLENTA

Somehow we think of Southern grits as more of a morning food than we do Italian polenta. Why is that? The differences between the two are rather slim, and both cook up into creamy comfort. So why not polenta for breakfast? This recipe relies on quick-cooking polenta, which means it's done in about five minutes. If you use a longer-cooking variety, you will need to increase the liquid and cooking time. I've worked a full 2 cups of milk into every pot, enriching it with protein and nutrients. The grated cheese and ham are flavorful window dressing.

1 ½ CUPS WATER

2 CUPS MILK

1 TEASPOON KOSHER SALT

⅔ CUP QUICK-COOKING POLENTA (SEE NOTE)

1 TABLESPOON BUTTER

½ CUP COARSELY GRATED SHARP CHEDDAR OR GRUYÈRE CHEESE

⅓ CUP CHOPPED HAM (ABOUT 3 THIN DELI SLICES)

FRESHLY GROUND BLACK PEPPER

1. Combine the water, milk, and salt in a medium saucepan over medium-high heat. Cook until it is just shy of a boil, keeping an eye on it so it doesn't boil over. Gradually add the polenta, whisking as you go. Lower the heat and simmer gently, stirring regularly, until the polenta absorbs the liquid and is tender, about 5 minutes. The polenta will thicken as it cools; feel free to add more water to thin it, if desired.

2. Remove the polenta from the heat. Add the butter and stir until it melts. Spoon the polenta into 4 serving bowls and top

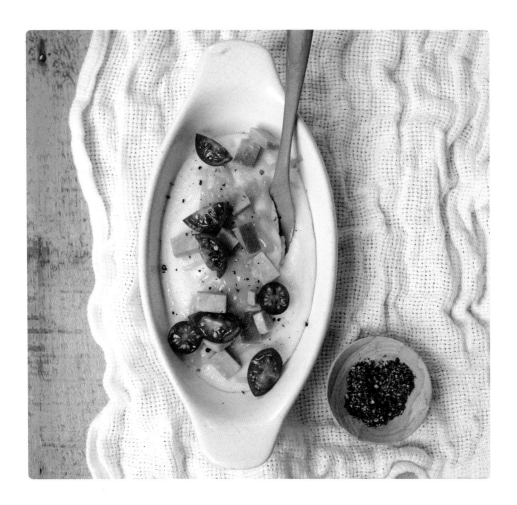

each with the cheese, ham, and a crack of black pepper. Serve immediately.

BOOST IT: Scatter a handful of halved cherry tomatoes over the polenta along with the ham and cheese.

MAKE AHEAD: Make polenta the night before and reheat it over low heat. Use a whisk to work out any lumps and add water as needed, ¼ cup at a time, until the polenta gets good and creamy again.

QUINOA BOWL WITH FALL FRUITS

Break out of your oatmeal rut and consider something new in that hot-cereal bowl: quinoa. Breakfast is actually my favorite meal for this teensy, protein-packed grain (which, technically, is not a grain at all but the seed of a plant in the amaranth family). Quinoa has a well-balanced amino acid profile and is especially rich in magnesium and iron. Make a fresh pot in the morning, or do it up as a side dish for dinner, relying on the leftovers to get you through breakfast. I like quinoa best doused with cold almond milk, roasted hazelnuts, and fall fruits. The reds and greens of apples, pears, and grapes make for a very pretty bowl.

1 CUP QUINOA

2 CUPS WATER

¼ TEASPOON KOSHER SALT

ALMOND MILK OR OTHER MILK OF YOUR CHOICE

1 CUP DICED PEAR, DICED APPLE, AND/OR HALVED GRAPES

¼ CUP CHOPPED ROASTED HAZELNUTS OR SLIVERED ALMONDS

HONEY OR PURE MAPLE SYRUP (OPTIONAL)

1. Check to see whether the quinoa has been prewashed. If so, there's no need to rinse it yourself. If not, put the quinoa into a fine-mesh sieve and rinse thoroughly over the sink to eliminate any bitterness. Allow to drain completely.

2. Transfer the quinoa to a medium saucepan and add the water and salt. Set the pan on the stove over high heat and bring to a boil. Lower the heat, cover with a lid, and simmer until the quinoa is tender, 15 to 18 minutes. Transfer the cooked quinoa to a fine-

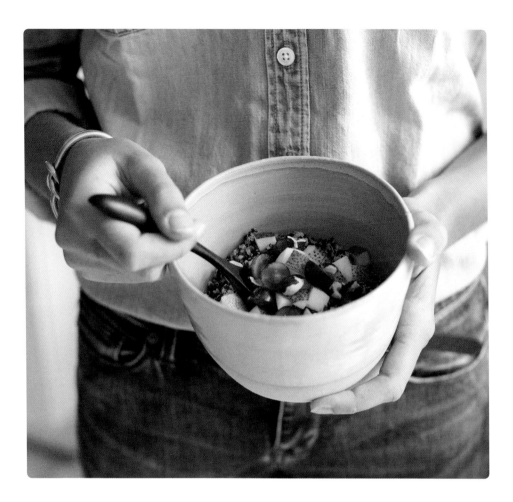

mesh sieve and give it a shake to drain off any remaining water.

3. To serve, spoon warm quinoa into bowls, add 1 to 2 tablespoons of milk, the diced fruit, and hazelnuts. Finish with a drizzle of honey or maple syrup, if desired.

MAKE AHEAD: You can cook the quinoa up to 3 days in advance and store it in the refrigerator. Reheat in the microwave, or add a couple teaspoons of water and warm on the stove over medium heat.

makes 4 or 5 servings

SLOW COOKER COCONUT RICE PUDDING

Rice pudding for breakfast sounds dreamy. And it is. Especially for the cook, because all it requires is stirring a handful of ingredients together in a slow cooker and flipping the "on" switch. Done. The brown rice cooks gently until it turns soft, fragrant from the coconut milk, and mildly sweet from the maple syrup. The coconut milk also adds richness that will have you double-dipping into your Crock-Pot. Any leftover pudding travels well in a lunch box and also makes a tasty after-school snack.

1 CUP BROWN BASMATI RICE

3 CUPS MILK

ONE 13.5-OUNCE CAN LIGHT COCONUT MILK

¼ CUP PURE MAPLE SYRUP

1 TEASPOON VANILLA EXTRACT

½ CUP RAISINS

1. Pour the rice into a fine-mesh sieve and rinse thoroughly over the sink. Allow to drain completely.

2. Transfer the rice to the slow cooker. Add the milk, coconut milk, maple syrup, and vanilla extract. Stir well. Put the lid on the slow cooker and set to low. Cook until most of the liquid is absorbed and the rice is very tender, about 4½ hours.

3. If a "skin" has formed across the top, simply mix it back into the pudding. Add the raisins and stir. Turn off the slow cooker. Serve warm or cold.

BOOST IT: Top the finished pudding with your favorite fresh berries.

MAKE AHEAD: This rice pudding can be made ahead of time and stored in the

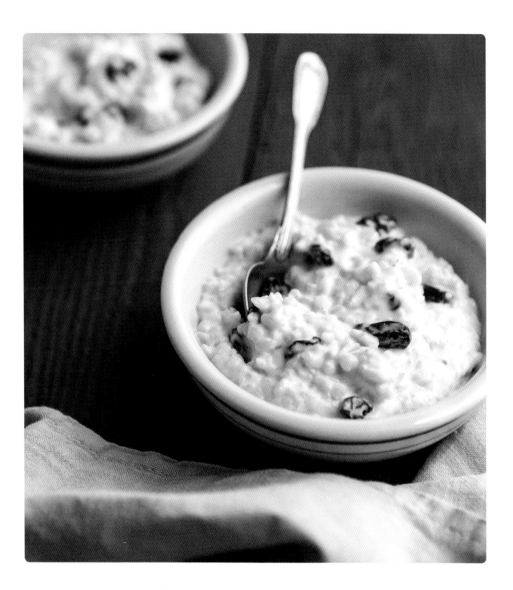

refrigerator for up to 3 days. It can be eaten cold or reheated. The rice will absorb more liquid as it cools, so feel free to add a little more milk, if desired.

MORNING FRIED RICE

The idea for this fried rice sprang from a conversation with fellow parent Dan Duane while we waited with our kids at the bus stop one day. It's an enormously flexible recipe that can be made with farro, spelt, or another sturdy grain in place of rice. It's even better when the rice is a day or so old, because it tends to crisp up and absorb the other flavors in the pan even better. Feel free to substitute any chopped leftover vegetables for the spinach. I use a little more egg than in typical fried rice because, well, it *is* breakfast, after all.

2 TABLESPOONS EXTRA-VIRGIN OLIVE OIL, DIVIDED

3 CUPS COOKED BROWN RICE, OR FARRO, SPELT, OR SORGHUM

½ CUP CHOPPED HAM

3 EGGS, LIGHTLY BEATEN

4 SCALLIONS, THINLY SLICED, WHITE AND LIGHT GREEN PARTS ONLY (ABOUT ⅓ CUP)

2 LARGE HANDFULS BABY SPINACH

1 TABLESPOON SEASONED RICE VINEGAR

1½ TEASPOONS SOY SAUCE

SRIRACHA OR OTHER HOT SAUCE (OPTIONAL)

1. Pour 1 tablespoon of the olive oil into a large skillet over medium-high heat. Add the rice and ham and cook, stirring regularly, until heated through, about 2 minutes (for a finished dish with a little more texture and crunch, cook an additional 1 to 2 minutes).

2. Push the rice far over to one side of the skillet. In the empty part of the pan, add ½ tablespoon of the remaining olive oil. Add the eggs and scramble them just until cooked through. Scoop up the eggs and put them on top of the rice. Pour the remaining

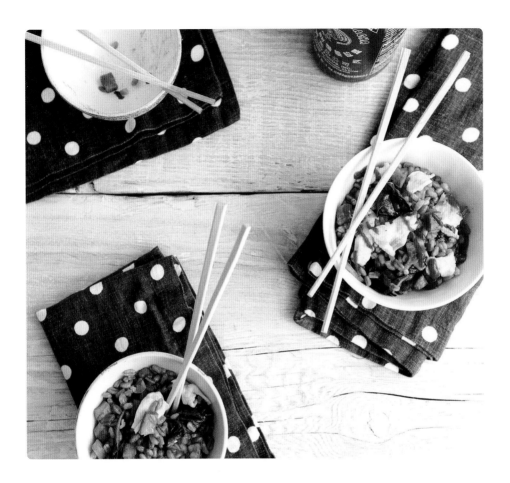

½ tablespoon of olive oil into the empty part of the pan and add the scallions. Sauté for about 1 minute to soften. Add the spinach and sauté just enough to wilt. Stir everything thoroughly together in the pan. Add the rice vinegar and soy sauce and stir

again. Serve with sriracha on the side, if desired.

BOOST IT: When you add the scallions to the pan, add a clove of thinly sliced garlic and/or one 1-inch piece of fresh ginger, finely chopped.

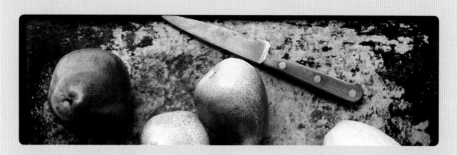

BREAKFAST-FRIENDLY FRUITS BY SEASON

Fresh, locally grown fruit is hard to beat, and buying what's in season often means more flavorful and more nutrient-packed produce. Many markets now specify where fruit was grown, giving you the option to choose, say, an apple that hails from fifty miles away instead of five thousand. One of the best ways to get your hands on excellent produce is to visit a farmers' market, where you can talk to the growers, taste the goods, and get your family engaged in farm-to-table eating. Here's how fruit stacks up by season, but keep in mind that this may vary based on where you live and that some fruits cross from one season into the next.

WINTER	SPRING	SUMMER	FALL
Mandarins	Guava	Peaches	Kiwifruits
Tangelos	Strawberries	Nectarines	Cranberries
Grapefruits	Cherries	Plums	Apples
Navel oranges	Rhubarb	Melons	Pomegranates
Blood oranges	Avocado	Raspberries	Persimmons
Pomelos	Apricots	Blackberries	Grapes
Kumquats	Apriums	Blueberries	Figs
			Pears

6

YOGURT AND FRUIT

yogurt and fruit go together like milk and cookies or peanut butter and jelly. That's something food companies figured out decades ago, when they started combining the two in little tubs to make fruit yogurt. Over the years, though, what was once relatively wholesome has evolved into something that often looks more like junk food than health food. In my own house, I used to buy fruit-flavored yogurt fairly regularly, but more recently I have gravitated toward plain. Any embellishing gets done in my own kitchen using simple ingredients.

In this chapter you'll find creative ways to play with yogurt. Some of the recipes are practically effortless, such as "Get Up and Go" Yogurt Cups (page 90) and Pretty Pomegranate Sundaes (page 97). Others don't need much hands-on time but do require a little patience in the cooking department, such as the Breakfast Baked Apples (page 100) and Honey Stewed Summer Fruit (page 94). You'll also find a couple of newfangled ideas, such as a yogurt bowl that's savory instead of sweet and a frozen pop that's bound to get any kid out of bed and to the breakfast table in no time.

"GET UP AND GO" YOGURT CUPS

Perhaps we all need to rethink our idea of what fast food really is. A tangerine? That's fast food. A peanut butter and banana sandwich? Check. And I'd argue that this yogurt cup is fast food too, because it's quick to make, economical, and easy to take on the road. I like to layer the ingredients in glass jars with lids and stow them in the fridge overnight. In the morning, grab one to enjoy at the kitchen table or tuck it into a backpack to eat at the bus stop. If you have a littler one who might not be as capable with a glass in her hand, make these in stainless steel or other reusable containers with lids.

⅓ CUP PLAIN GREEK YOGURT

⅓ CUP VANILLA YOGURT

⅓ CUP BLUEBERRIES, RASPBERRIES, OR BLACKBERRIES

¼ CUP GRANOLA

1 TABLESPOON TOASTED COCONUT CHIPS

1. In a jelly jar or drinking glass, stir together the Greek and vanilla yogurts with a small spoon. Top with the berries, granola, and coconut chips, in that order.

   BOOST IT: Add a few teaspoons of hemp or chia seeds along with the granola.
   ADAPT IT: This recipe calls for equal parts plain and sweetened yogurt, which cuts down on the sugar. If your kids are unaccustomed to plain yogurt, it may take their palates time to adjust. Try using a little more vanilla yogurt at first, and then scale back over time as they get used to the flavor being more tangy than sweet.
   MAKE AHEAD: Yogurt cups can be made the night before. Cover with a jar lid or plastic wrap and store in the fridge.

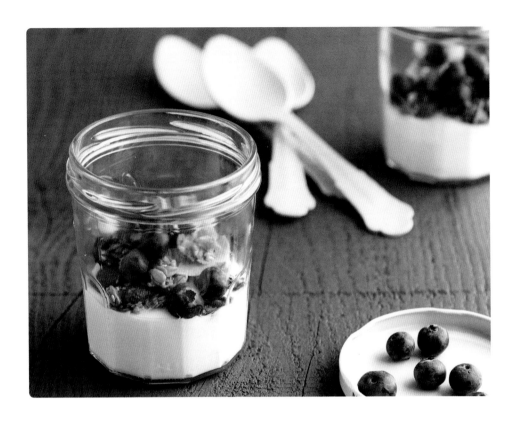

DON'T OVERLOOK FROZEN FRUIT

TIP

Fresh local produce year-round may be a reality for folks in California and Florida, but not for those in places where below-zero temperatures make an inhospitable environment for farms and gardens, to say the least. Thankfully, frozen fruit stacks up really well nutritionally, because it goes into the deep freeze at the peak of ripeness, soon after harvesting, which keeps vitamins, minerals, and fiber largely intact. It also means you have fruit at your fingertips, already washed, prepped, and recipe-ready.

RASPBERRY CHIA YOGURT POPS

Pops for breakfast? Really? That's what my kids said when I began tinkering with the idea. But guess what? They've become a favorite, most especially among my older kids, who don't always want to take time for something so mundane as eating. They grab one as they walk out the door, getting at least a little something into their bellies before the day begins. Because they aren't sweetened as much as standard pops, I like to use whole-milk yogurt instead of reduced fat because it adds richness to offset the yogurt's tang. The chia seeds help the raspberry syrup gel quickly and add nourishment to these colorful pops.

1 CUP FRESH OR FROZEN RASPBERRIES

1½ TABLESPOONS HONEY

1 TABLESPOON CHIA SEEDS

1½ CUP VANILLA YOGURT (I PREFER WHOLE-MILK YOGURT HERE)

½ CUP PLAIN GREEK YOGURT

1. Put the raspberries and honey into a small saucepan over medium heat. As the berries warm and the honey melts, give it a stir with a fork. Continue to cook, stirring regularly and mashing the raspberries with the fork. After about 3 minutes, the berries will be melted and the liquid will begin to boil. Once it boils, remove the pan from the heat, add the chia seeds, and stir. Put the pan into the fridge to cool completely, about 1 hour.

2. Put the vanilla yogurt and Greek yogurt into a medium bowl, ideally one with a spout for pouring, and stir with a whisk until smooth and well combined. Spoon the chilled raspberry sauce over the yogurt and stir gently several times

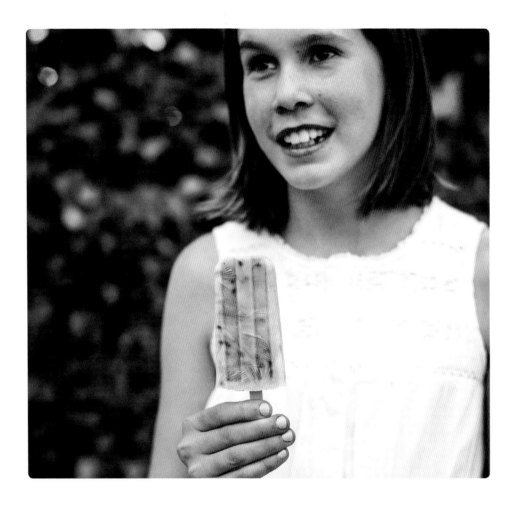

to mix it into the yogurt. It doesn't need to be completely incorporated, just stirred enough so that the raspberries are distributed throughout.

3. Pour the yogurt mixture into pop molds and freeze.

BOOST IT: Stir as much as 1 cup of your favorite granola into the yogurt mixture before pouring into pop molds.

makes 4 servings

HONEY STEWED SUMMER FRUIT

I learned to make this warm and luscious fruit dish from my sister Annie, who spends time most summers in France with her in-laws. There, she watches the morning ritual of her mother-in-law, who stews a big pot of whatever fruit happens to be in season into a tender compote to spoon over yogurt for breakfast. As much as I love ripe-off-the-tree plums, peaches, and nectarines, gently cooking these fruits in their own juices along with a touch of honey renders them something different altogether: comforting, both sweet and tangy, and soft. This dish has become my favorite way to begin the day during the summer months, when stone fruits are at their peak. It's also an excellent topping for waffles, pancakes, and even ordinary toast.

1 POUND PEACHES, NECTARINES, OR PLUMS

2 TABLESPOONS WATER

2 TABLESPOONS HONEY

PLAIN GREEK OR REGULAR YOGURT, FOR SERVING

1. Cut the fruit in half and remove the pits. Cut the halves into wedges that are 1 to 1½ inches wide.
2. Put the water and honey into a medium saucepan over high heat. Cook, stirring continuously, until the honey melts into the water, about 30 seconds. Add the fruit, stir, and let the mixture come to a boil. Drop the heat to low, cover with a lid, and cook, stirring occasionally, until the fruit is very soft but hasn't completely lost its shape, about 15 minutes. The cooking time will vary depending on the ripeness and size of the fruits. Remove from the heat.

3. To serve, spoon the warm fruit and some of its juices over plain yogurt.

ADAPT IT: When rhubarb is in season, use it in place of the stone fruit. Cut the stalks into 1-inch lengths and increase the amount of honey because rhubarb lacks the natural sweetness of stone fruits.

MAKE AHEAD: This is so delicious, you may find you go through a batch pretty quickly. Luckily, the recipe can be doubled easily, and leftovers can be stored in an airtight container in the fridge for up to 5 days.

YOGURT: SHOULD YOU GO GREEK?

Greek yogurt doesn't belong exclusively to the Greeks. A number of countries favor this style of yogurt, in which the whey is strained off to create a supremely creamy, thick consistency. The process results in a yogurt that has two times the protein and fewer carbohydrates than its unstrained counterpart. Is there a downside? If you're looking to yogurt as a calcium source, you should know that Greek yogurt has significantly less than other yogurt.

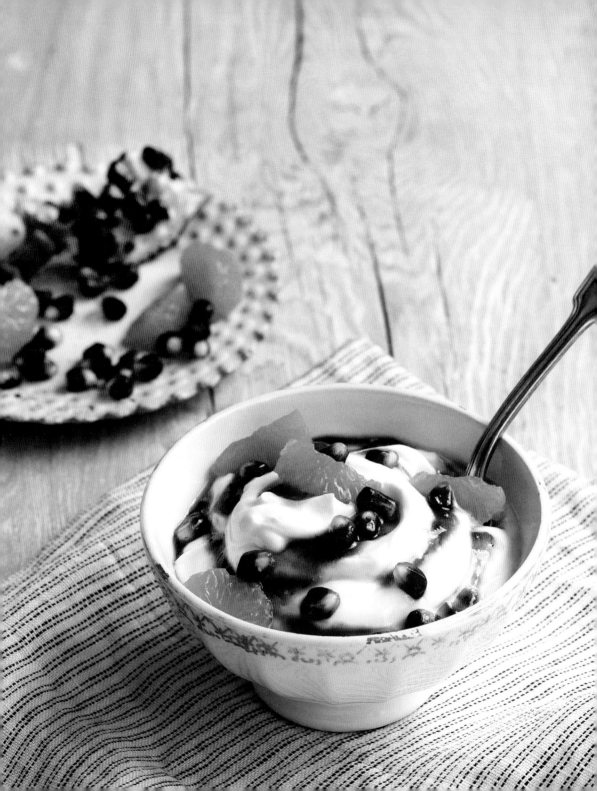

PRETTY POMEGRANATE SUNDAES

Children, like all of us, respond to smart marketing. A study at Cornell University found that renaming carrots to make them sound more appealing doubled their consumption in school cafeterias. I'm applying that same logic to this recipe, by naming it a sundae. It's certainly tasty enough, with plenty of eye appeal. You can even pull out an ice cream scoop and spoon the yogurt into dessert dishes instead of cereal bowls. Sundaes for breakfast? Your kids will think you're a rock star.

1 ½ CUPS PLAIN GREEK YOGURT

1 TO 2 TABLESPOONS STRAWBERRY JAM

3 SMALL SEEDLESS TANGERINES, PEELED

⅓ CUP POMEGRANATE SEEDS (SEE NOTE)

1. Divide the yogurt between 2 small bowls or ice cream dishes.
2. Put the jam in a small ramekin or glass bowl and microwave on high for 10 seconds. Pour the jam over the yogurt.
3. Lay the tangerines on their sides and use a serrated knife to cut them into ½-inch-thick slices. Pull the segments apart and scatter over the yogurt. Top with the pomegranate seeds.

Note: You will save time by buying pomegranate seeds rather than a whole pomegranate that you will need to seed yourself. The seeds are often sold in the supermarket produce section near other prepared fruits and vegetables.

BOOST IT: Top each sundae with 1 tablespoon of toasted slivered almonds.

MAKE AHEAD: Make these up to a day in advance, cover with plastic wrap, and refrigerate overnight.

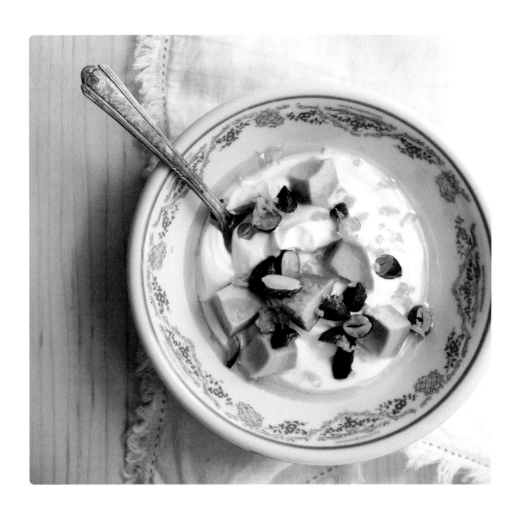

STIR IN THE WHEY

TIP

The liquid that floats to the top of yogurt is simply whey that's separated from the solids. It's tangy and has a small amount of protein, so just stir it right back in.

SAVORY YOGURT BOWLS

Hang on to your hats, people. This recipe may strike you as a little strange, but do as I did when my friend Liz told me about her savory breakfast bowls: don't knock it till you try it. If you consider that much of the world eats yogurt with salt and spices (think Indian raita and Greek tzatziki), you'll realize that we're just a little late to the game. The yogurt here is perfumed with lemon zest and topped with creamy avocado and toasted almonds. Talk about healthy fats! It's not a big breakfast but delivers a nutrient-dense package that will have everyone bright eyed and bushy tailed all morning long.

1 CUP PLAIN GREEK YOGURT

1 TEASPOON EXTRA-VIRGIN OLIVE OIL

SALT

½ LEMON

½ LARGE RIPE AVOCADO, CUT INTO SMALL CUBES

⅓ CUP CHOPPED OR SLIVERED TOASTED ALMONDS

1. Spoon the yogurt into 2 small serving bowls, such as cereal bowls. Drizzle the olive oil over the 2 bowls and add a tiny pinch of salt to each. Zest enough lemon rind over the yogurt so that it looks like a little shower of lemon "snow" on top. Stir well. Top with the avocado and a few drops of fresh lemon juice. Sprinkle a tiny pinch of salt over the avocado and then top with the almonds.

BOOST IT: This recipe is extra tasty with zest from a Meyer lemon. It's also particularly good if you toast the almonds yourself and add them to the yogurt while they are still warm from the oven.

makes 4 servings

BREAKFAST BAKED APPLES

Wander into the kitchen to get your coffee brewing, and while you're there, take a few minutes (five, tops) to assemble these apples and get them bubbling in the oven. By the time your crew is up, dressed, and sitting at the table, you'll have a warm, nourishing, tangy apple waiting for them. Top each one with yogurt and a drizzle of maple syrup, and you'll have a breakfast that will hold off hunger until noon. Bake some extra apples and stow them in the fridge for an afternoon snack, simple dessert, or breakfast the next day. For littler appetites, half an apple will suffice.

4 MEDIUM PINK LADY APPLES OR OTHER COOKING APPLES OF YOUR CHOICE

½ CUP GRANOLA

2 TEASPOONS PURE MAPLE SYRUP, PLUS MORE FOR SERVING

1 TABLESPOON BUTTER, CUT INTO 4 PIECES

PLAIN YOGURT, FOR SERVING

1. Preheat the oven or toaster oven to 400°F. Line the bottom of an 8 × 8-inch baking pan with parchment paper (be sure the pan fits in the toaster oven, if using).

2. Remove the cores from the apples using an apple corer or melon baller and set the apples upright in the baking pan. Fill the cavity of each apple with the granola, packing it down firmly with your thumb until it's level with the top of the apple. Pour maple syrup slowly onto the granola in each apple, and put a piece of butter on top.

3. Bake the apples for 30 to 40 minutes, until they're quite tender and begin to crack and ooze their juices. Cooking time will vary depending on the size and variety of the apples.

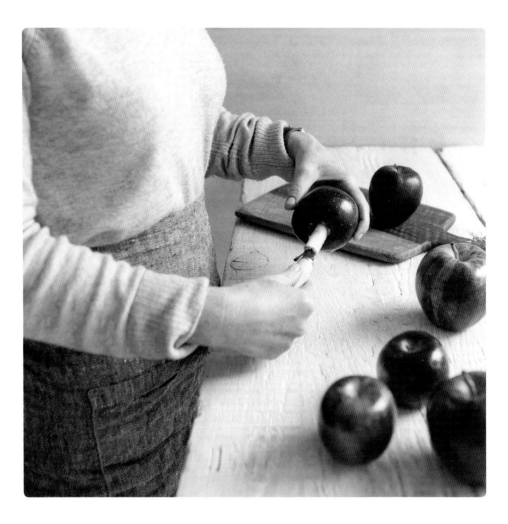

4. Serve each apple in a shallow bowl topped with a generous spoonful of yogurt and a drizzle of maple syrup.

MAKE AHEAD: Assemble the apples the night before and bake them in the morning. Once baked, apples will keep in the fridge in a covered container for up to 3 days.

ANATOMY OF A SUCCESSFUL BREAKFAST SANDWICH

Sandwich making is more art than science, but a handful of ground rules can up your game when creating these handheld classics.

THE BREAD: Bread is everything when it comes to a scrumptious sandwich. Get your hands on a loaf from a good bakery or bread shop if you can; it's likely to be superior to mainstream brands. That said, mediocre bread can be improved immensely after a few minutes in the toaster. Also, the ratio of bread to filling is key. Too much bread, and what's inside gets buried. Too skimpy a slice, and the whole thing falls apart. Dense and hearty breads hold up well when thin, while more tender loaves lend themselves to thicker slices.

THE SPREAD: A tasty shmear of anything from salty butter to herbed cream cheese can add flavor and creaminess and, in some cases, provide a barrier so bread won't go soggy. Be sure to coat the entire surface so that every bite will be packed with flavor.

THE FILLINGS: The sky's the limit for what makes a satisfying filling. Eggs are the foundation for breakfast sandwiches the world over, but no need to stop there. Keep in mind that you want your sandwich to hold you through morning, so look for protein-rich fixings, and think about adding fruits, vegetables, and other nourishing goodies. Super-moist ingredients, such as tomatoes and soft fruits, should be tucked in the center so your bread will stay nice and dry.

THE FLAVORS: The creative part is layering on ingredients that cover the whole flavor spectrum: sweet, sour, salty, tangy, spicy, and aromatic. Here's where you'll want to rifle through the fridge for fresh herbs, pickled jalapeños, basil pesto, a favorite jam, capers, chile sauce, or whatever else strikes your fancy.

7
SANDWICHES AND WRAPS

sandwiches aren't just for lunch anymore. In fact, sandwiches are among the top ten breakfast foods Americans buy when eating out. So why not choose them when eating in too? Everything that makes them appealing at midday makes them just as suitable first thing in the morning: they're easy to prepare, filling, and, when done right, nutritionally well balanced. Ditto for wraps, which are really just sandwiches dressed in a slightly different uniform.

I'm smitten with this sort of portable breakfast. While I have a few classics in this chapter, I've gone rogue with a lot of them, tinkering with the traditional and expanding the notion of what a breakfast sandwich really is. You'll find a PB&J made in a waffle iron, a BLT on a bagel, and a delicate tea sandwich with fresh strawberries in place of more traditional fixings.

My aim with these recipes is to emphasize whole grain breads, work in plenty of fruits and vegetables, include a source or two of protein, keep the portion sizes just right, and do it all in mega-tasty edible packages.

Eat these sandwiches and wraps at the kitchen table, or pack them up and take them to go. You'll be well fueled until the lunch hour rolls around, when, who knows, you may be sitting down to another sandwich.

DRIVE-THROUGH EGG SANDWICH

It's much better to drive through your kitchen than a fast-food place to pick up breakfast, especially when there's an egg sandwich as tasty as this one. Everything gets done in one pan, including toasting the English muffin, which crisps up on the outside while the cheese melts on the inside. This is just the thing to wrap up in parchment and hand off to your child, who may not even notice you've tucked some spinach in the center.

2 CANADIAN BACON SLICES

2 WHOLE GRAIN ENGLISH MUFFINS, SPLIT IN HALF

SMALL HANDFUL BABY SPINACH (ABOUT ½ CUP, GENTLY PACKED)

2 THIN SLICES SHARP CHEDDAR CHEESE

2 TEASPOONS EXTRA-VIRGIN OLIVE OIL, DIVIDED

2 LARGE EGGS

PINCH OF SALT

FRESHLY GROUND BLACK PEPPER

1. Lay 1 slice of Canadian bacon on the bottom half of each English muffin. Top with spinach, followed by cheese. Set aside.

2. Heat 1 teaspoon of the oil in a medium cast iron or nonstick skillet over medium-high heat. Crack the eggs into the skillet and add a pinch of salt and a few cracks of pepper. Cook for 2 minutes. Flip the eggs over and cook another 30 seconds for a soft-cooked egg, or until firm to the touch for a fully cooked yolk. Use a spatula to transfer the eggs onto the top of the spinach and cheese. Cover with the English muffin tops.

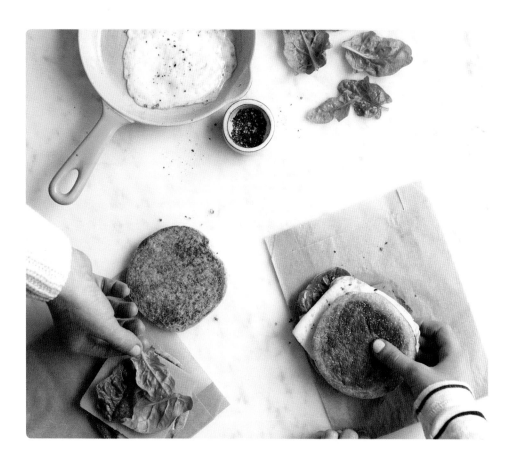

3. Pour the remaining 1 teaspoon of oil into the pan, swirl to coat the bottom, and raise the heat to high. Set the sandwiches in the pan and cook until the English muffins are brown and a little crispy on the bottom (don't worry if a little yolk oozes out). Turn the sandwiches over and cook until the cheese is melted and the muffins are evenly browned on the second side.

ADAPT IT: This recipe can be adjusted in many ways. Use a different cheese, leave out the Canadian bacon, or swap a sliced tomato for the spinach.

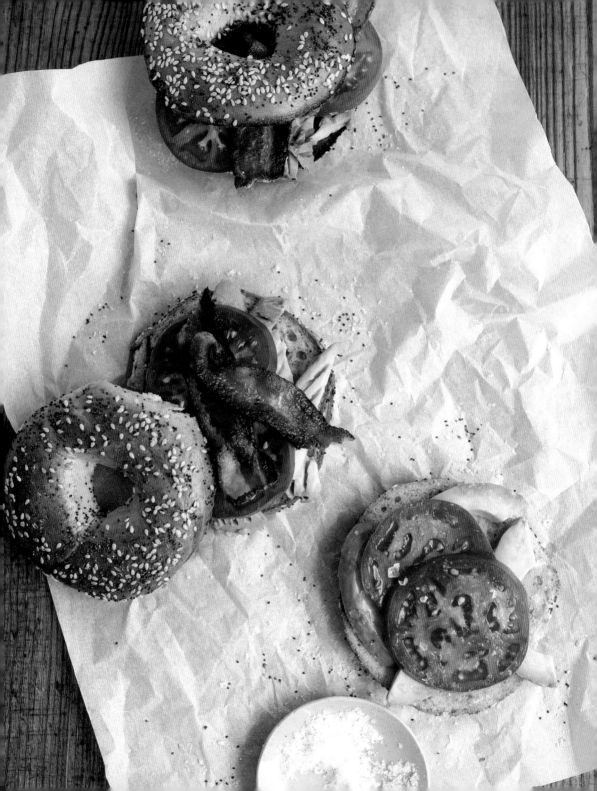

makes 3 sandwiches

GOOD MORNING BLT

Vegetarians notwithstanding, everyone I know loves a BLT. So why wait until lunch to enjoy one, especially when bacon and, in this case, bagels are traditional morning foods? These BLTs are more healthful than most because they're lighter on the bacon, they call for whole grain bagels, and they rely on avocado instead of mayonnaise for a creamy spread. The key to making bagels work well for sandwiches is to cut them into thin rounds instead of halves; this way the bread won't overwhelm the filling. A little squeeze of lemon over the top does wonders to brighten the flavor, so don't skip this step.

2 WHOLE GRAIN "EVERYTHING" BAGELS (NOT PRE-SLICED)

1 MEDIUM RIPE AVOCADO

½ LEMON

PINCH OF SALT

1 LARGE RIPE TOMATO

6 COOKED BACON SLICES

HANDFUL OF BABY LETTUCE

1. Using a serrated knife, carefully cut each of the bagels into three rounds instead of in half. This will make 6 bagel slices, enough for 3 sandwiches. Lightly toast the slices in the toaster.

2. Scoop out the flesh of the avocado and divide evenly among 3 of the bagel slices, smashing it down with a fork. Gently squeeze a little lemon juice over the avocado, followed by a pinch of salt. Cut three ¼-inch-thick slices of tomato. Lay the tomato slices on top of the avocado. Tear the cooked bacon slices in half and lay on top of

each tomato slice. Place the baby lettuce on top of the bacon, evenly distributing it among the sandwiches, and top with the 3 remaining bagel slices.

MAKE AHEAD: Cook the bacon a day in advance, then wrap it up and store in the fridge until ready to use.

IS BACON SO BAD?

Many of us have a love-hate relationship with bacon. We love its salty, crispy goodness; we hate that it's not so good for us. Does that mean bacon should be banned? Should other cured meats, such as prosciutto, ham, and sausage, for that matter? Not necessarily. Sure, bacon is a source of saturated fat. And yes, it's processed with nitrates, a known carcinogen. But it also packs a whole lot of flavor into a little package. If it's eaten in reasonable portions as part of a healthy diet, I don't see a problem with a bit of bacon. For myself, I look for brands labeled "uncured," which means the nitrates come from a natural source instead of a chemical one. I also try to keep the serving size to a slice or two (not the entire pound!), and I blot the cooked slices with a paper towel to remove excess fat before serving.

makes 1 sandwich

OOZY PEAR AND GRUYÈRE PANINI

The inspiration for this recipe comes from my first job. I worked at a gourmet food shop, and among my duties was making fancy sandwiches, including a cheese and pear chutney number. I still love the combination of creamy cheese and sweet pear, and so do my kids. Yours might love this sandwich too, especially when done up in a panini press. The stove-top method described here works great, too.

ONE 5-INCH SEGMENT OF A FRENCH BAGUETTE

ENOUGH THIN SLICES OF GRUYÈRE CHEESE TO COVER THE BOTTOM HALF OF THE BAGUETTE TWICE

ENOUGH ¼-INCH-THICK SLICES OF PEAR TO COVER THE BOTTOM HALF OF THE BAGUETTE ONCE

1 TEASPOON EXTRA-VIRGIN OLIVE OIL

1. Cut the baguette in half lengthwise. Cover the bottom half of the baguette with 1 layer of Gruyère, 1 layer of pear, and a second layer of Gruyère. Cover with the top of the baguette.

2. Set a medium skillet over medium heat. Add the olive oil and swirl the pan to coat the bottom. Place the sandwich in the pan and place your heaviest pot on top. Press down on the pot very firmly for a few seconds. Cook the sandwich with the pot on top until the bottom of the sandwich is lightly browned and crispy, about 2 minutes. Flip the sandwich over and return the pot to the top of the sandwich. Press down on the pot for a few more seconds and cook the sandwich until the second side is brown and the cheese is melted, about 2 minutes more. Cut in half and serve.

BOOST IT: Tuck a handful of arugula between the layers of cheese and pear.

ADAPT IT: Swap pear for apple.

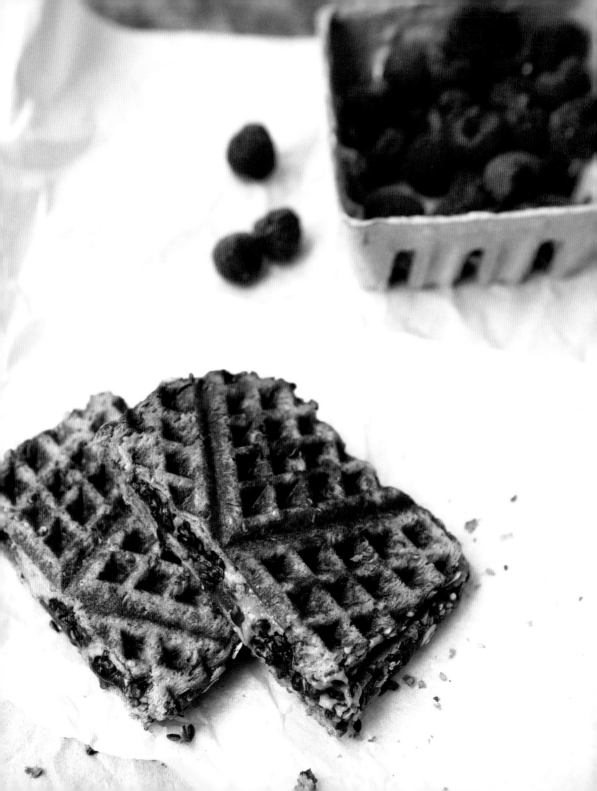

PEANUT BUTTER RASPBERRY WAFFLE IRON SANDWICH

This recipe gives the iconic PB&J the breakfast treatment by toasting it in a waffle iron, which acts something like a panini press. The result is a sandwich that's crispy on the outside and deliciously warm on the inside. I've swapped out the jam here and used fresh raspberries instead, which means less sugar and a brighter, tangier fruit flavor. The sandwich is a good one to take on the go, either for breakfast or wrapped up and tucked into a lunch box.

2 SLICES WHOLE GRAIN SANDWICH BREAD

1 ½ TABLESPOONS UNSWEETENED PEANUT BUTTER

6 RASPBERRIES

1. Preheat your waffle iron.
2. Lay the sandwich bread on your work surface. Spread the peanut butter evenly over the top of both slices. Lay the raspberries on 1 slice of bread, distributing them evenly. Cover with the remaining slice of bread, keeping the peanut butter on the inside.
3. Grease the waffle iron with oil or non-stick cooking spray. Put the sandwich into the waffle iron and close. Press down firmly on the lid. (It may not close completely.) Cook until the bread is brown and crispy. Cut in half and serve.

ADAPT IT: Any nut, seed, or soy butter will work in place of the peanut butter.

makes 1 sandwich

FRENCH KIDS' BREAKFAST BAGUETTE

Lest you think I'm crazy for suggesting a chocolate sandwich for breakfast, consider this: dark chocolate chips have less sugar by weight than your typical fruit preserves. Let's not forget about the healthful antioxidants in that dark chocolate, either. Nevertheless, I consider this more of a "sometimes treat" than an everyday breakfast, even if chocolate sandwiches are nearly as common in France as PB&Js are here.

ONE 4-INCH-LONG SEGMENT OF A FRENCH BAGUETTE (IDEALLY WHOLE GRAIN)

2 TABLESPOONS DARK CHOCOLATE CHIPS

½ SMALL BANANA

1. Preheat the oven or toaster oven to 350°F.
2. Split the baguette in half lengthwise. Scatter the chocolate chips over the bottom half of the baguette. Put the baguette half into the oven or toaster oven (directly on the rack is OK) and heat until the chocolate softens enough to spread, about 2 minutes. Remove the baguette from the oven and use a knife to spread the chocolate across the surface.
3. Cut the banana into ¼-inch-thick rounds and place on top of the chocolate in a single layer. Cover with the top half of the baguette.

BOOST IT: Spread up to 1 tablespoon of peanut butter or other nut or seed butter of your choice inside the top half of the baguette before covering the sandwich.

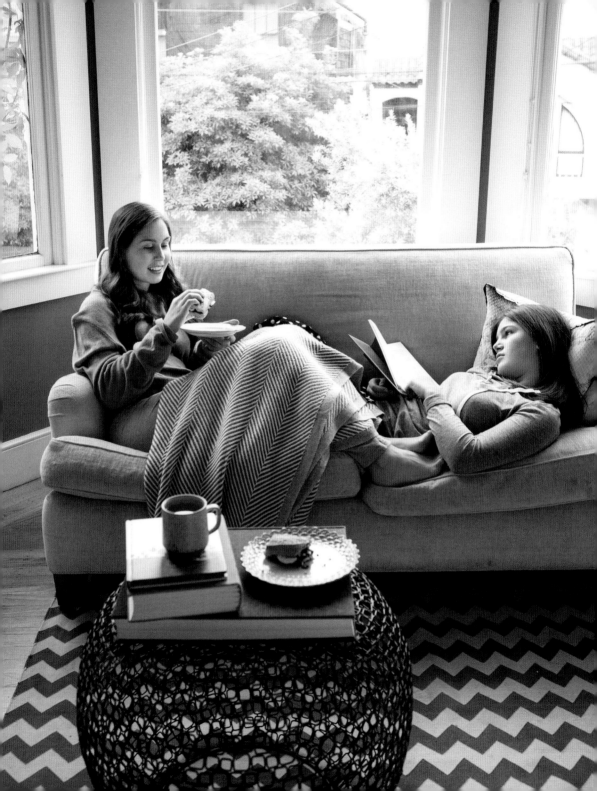

QUICK FIX

8 EASY IDEAS FOR SANDWICHES AND WRAPS

1. Spread hummus on two pieces of sandwich bread and layer cucumber slices between them. Cut in half.

2. Coat one side of a whole grain tortilla with nut, seed, or peanut butter, scatter a tablespoon of raisins over it, and roll up.

3. Make a baguette sandwich with mozzarella, tomato slices, and basil pesto.

4. Sprinkle baby kale and grated cheese over lavash bread, microwave for 45 seconds, and fold in half.

5. Put a shmear of cream cheese followed by a layer of your favorite jam on the halves of a toasted whole grain English muffin.

6. Mash half of an avocado over a slice of whole grain toast. Sprinkle with salt and lemon juice and top with baby greens and a second slice of toast.

7. Slice a hard-boiled egg and tuck it into a warm pita pocket. Add salt, black pepper, and a drizzle of olive oil.

8. Spread apple butter over a slice of whole grain raisin toast and layer Cheddar slices and apple slices on top. Cover with a second slice of toast.

STRAWBERRY RICOTTA TEA SANDWICH

The quality of your ingredients will make or break this delicate yet filling tea sandwich. Make it in spring or summer when fresh, ripe strawberries are in season, and go the extra mile to get your hands on a good ricotta cheese. Look for one made with little more than milk, an acid or starter, and salt. Bellweather Farms and Calabro are two of my favorite brands that have fairly wide distribution. If you've never had ricotta like this before, you're in for a treat.

2 SLICES SOFT WHOLE GRAIN BREAD, WITH CRUSTS CUT OFF

3 TABLESPOONS FRESH RICOTTA CHEESE

1 LEMON

4 MEDIUM STRAWBERRIES, CUT INTO ¼-INCH SLICES

1 TEASPOON HONEY

1. Lightly toast the bread. Spread the ricotta over one side of both slices of toast. Use a zester or fine grater to zest a very light shower of lemon peel over the ricotta. Arrange the sliced strawberries in a layer over the ricotta on one slice of the toast (a little bit of overlap is OK). Drizzle the honey over the strawberries. Cover with the remaining toast, keeping the ricotta on the inside. Cut in half.

ADAPT IT: Use 2 tablespoons of whipped cream cheese in place of the ricotta.

NUTTY BANANA BITES

This is one of those breakfast recipes to keep in your back pocket for when you're short on time and the pantry is emptied of all but the most basic ingredients. It's quick to make and can be taken on the road. When they're in season and on hand, use berries instead of banana, scattering them over the tortilla and then rolling them snug inside.

1 WHOLE GRAIN FLOUR TORTILLA

1 ½ TABLESPOONS NUT, PEANUT, OR SUNFLOWER BUTTER

1 MEDIUM BANANA

1. Lay the tortilla on your work surface. Spread the nut butter over the tortilla to just shy of the edge. Place the whole banana on top of the tortilla near the edge closest to you. (The banana's ends should be pointing left and right.) Roll the banana up completely in the tortilla. Cut the roll crosswise into 6 rounds.

   BOOST IT: Scatter 1 tablespoon of sunflower seeds over the nut butter before adding the banana.
   ADAPT IT: Leave out the banana and make this into a simple nut-butter roll-up.

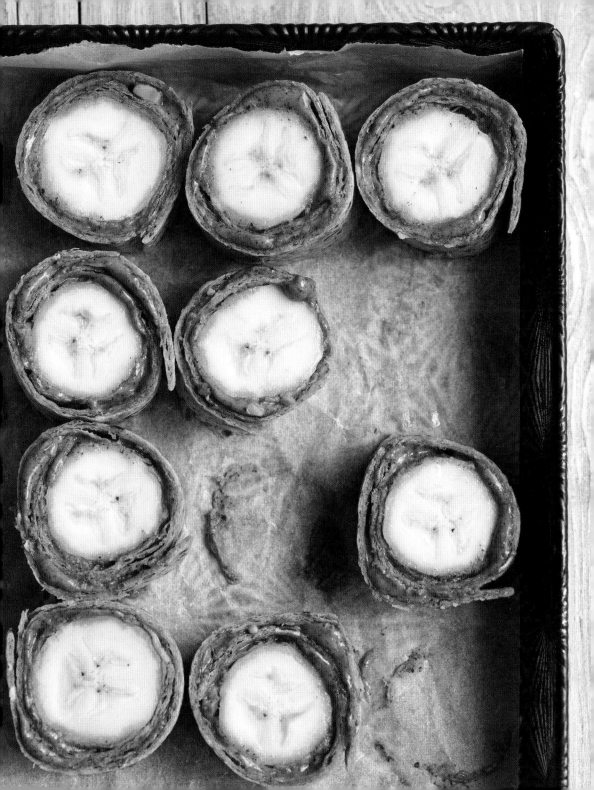

TEX MEX TOFU WRAPS

My kids, who claim to not be particularly fond of tofu, love this wrap. Warmed in olive oil with crunchy carrots, flavorful salsa, and that little bit of cheese, it's just plain tasty. Tofu is a protein-rich breakfast alternative to eggs that's both afford-able and nourishing. If you take a couple shortcuts here—buying preshredded carrots and pregrated cheese—you can have these ready to eat in minutes.

1½ TEASPOONS EXTRA-VIRGIN OLIVE OIL

8 OUNCES FIRM TOFU, DRAINED WELL

¾ CUP COARSELY SHREDDED CARROTS (SEE NOTE)

2 TABLESPOONS MEXICAN SALSA, PLUS MORE IF DESIRED

¼ TEASPOON KOSHER SALT

FOUR 8-INCH WHOLE GRAIN FLOUR TORTILLAS

⅓ CUP COARSELY GRATED MONTEREY JACK OR CHEDDAR CHEESE

1. Set a medium skillet over medium heat. Add the oil and swirl the pan to coat the bottom. Crumble the tofu into the pan with your hands. Add the carrots and heat, stirring gently, until they are warmed through and slightly tender, about 2 minutes. Add the salsa and salt, stir again, and remove from heat.

2. While the tofu and carrots are cook-ing, place the tortillas on a work sur-face. Divide the cheese among the tortillas and distribute evenly over the top. Microwave the cheese-covered tortillas—1 or 2 at a time—on high for 30 to 40 seconds, until the cheese is melted and the tortillas are warm.

3. Spoon the tofu mixture into the center of each tortilla. Add more salsa, if de-sired. Fold up "burrito style" and serve.

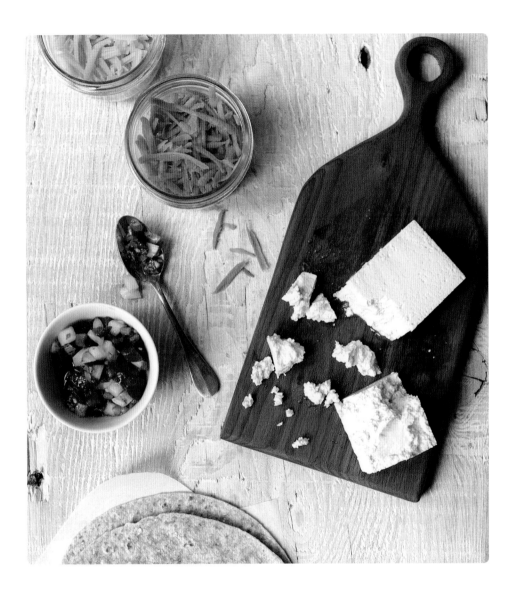

ADAPT IT: Substitute another shredded vegetable for the carrots, such as zucchini, sweet potato, or winter squash, or leave them out.

CHEESY GREENS QUESADILLA

In a culture that makes it so very convenient to eat an unhealthy diet, I'm always looking for ways that make it easy to eat a healthy one. One trick is to keep the fridge stocked with grab-and-go vegetables placed right at eye level. I almost always have a bag of kale, spinach, arugula, collards, or other favorite greens that are washed, stemmed, chopped, and ready to use. Nothing could be easier than adding a handful of greens to a quesadilla and calling it breakfast.

ONE 8-INCH WHOLE GRAIN FLOUR TORTILLA

⅓ CUP COARSELY GRATED HAVARTI OR OTHER GRATED CHEESE OF YOUR CHOICE

½ GENTLY PACKED CUP BABY KALE OR BABY SPINACH

1 TEASPOON EXTRA-VIRGIN OLIVE OIL

1. Lay the tortilla on a work surface and cover one half of it with half of the cheese. Top the cheese with the kale, followed by the remaining cheese. Fold the plain half of the tortilla over the cheese to form a half moon.

2. Set a medium skillet over medium-high heat. Add the olive oil and swirl the pan to coat the bottom. Place the folded tortilla into the pan and cook until brown and crisp on the bottom. Use a spatula to flip it over and cook the second side until browned and the cheese is melted.

3. Remove the quesadilla from the pan, cut into 4 wedges, and serve.

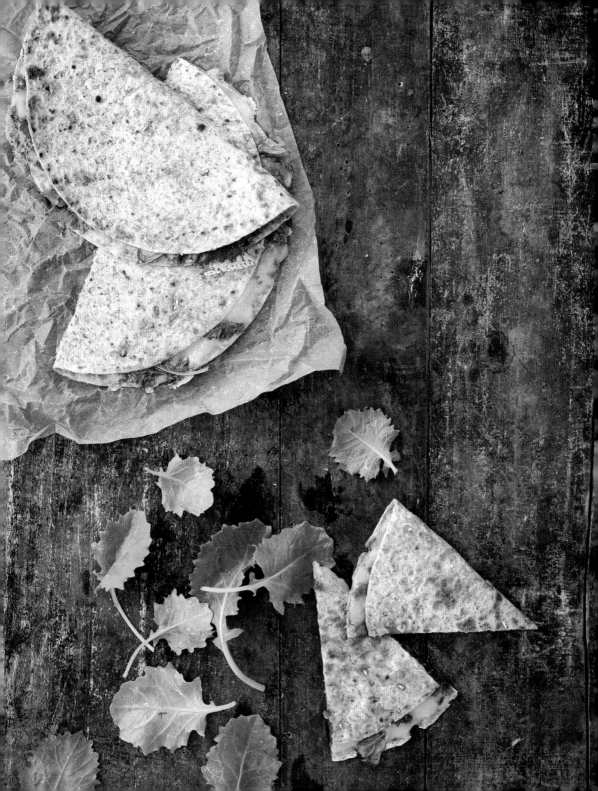

FREEZER-FRIENDLY BREAKFAST BURRITOS

A flavor bomb in a tidy, highly portable package—that's what these are. Filled with eggs, zucchini, cheese, beans, and just enough Spanish chorizo to pack some heat and smoke, they're immensely satisfying—a home run, according to my family. What makes these workable for weekdays is that you can prep them ahead and stow them in the fridge or freezer. They keep beautifully. If you can't get your hands on chorizo, cooked andouille sausage or Polish kielbasa will do the job as well.

2 TEASPOONS EXTRA-VIRGIN OLIVE OIL

¾ CUP DICED ZUCCHINI (¼-INCH DICE—ABOUT 1 SMALL ZUCCHINI)

4 EGGS, LIGHTLY BEATEN

HEAPING ½ CUP DICED COOKED SPANISH CHORIZO (¼-INCH DICE)

½ CUP COOKED BLACK BEANS, DRAINED AND RINSED

FOUR 8-INCH FLOUR TORTILLAS

¾ CUP COARSELY GRATED MONTEREY JACK CHEESE

1 TABLESPOON PLUS 1 TEASPOON MEXICAN SALSA

1. Set a large skillet over medium-high heat. Add the oil and swirl the pan to coat the bottom. Add the zucchini and sauté until just tender, 1 to 2 minutes. Lower the heat to medium-low and add the eggs. Use a rubber spatula to gently scramble the eggs with the zucchini until the eggs are nearly cooked. Remove the pan from heat, add the chorizo and black beans, and stir gently, allowing the heat of the pan to warm them through.

2. Lay the tortillas on a work surface and divide the cheese evenly among

them. Distribute the cheese evenly over the top, to about 1 inch shy of the edge. Microwave the cheese-covered tortillas—1 or 2 at a time—on high for 30 to 40 seconds, until the cheese is melted and the tortillas are warm.

3. Spoon a quarter of the egg mixture into the center of each tortilla. Roll up "burrito-style" and serve.

ADAPT IT: Use diced ham in place of the chorizo, and substitute practically any vegetable for the zucchini. Heartier vegetables will take longer to cook.

MAKE AHEAD: These burritos freeze well, which makes this a good recipe to double and store for future meals. To freeze, allow the burritos to cool completely, then wrap each one individually in plastic wrap. Store in a resealable plastic bag with the air pressed out. To reheat, defrost in the refrigerator overnight. Remove plastic wrap and heat in the microwave on high until warmed through, about 45 seconds.

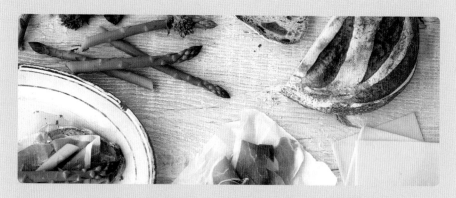

THE ART OF ARTISAN TOAST

Who knew toast would go trendy, but so it has: simple slices are topping four dollars a pop in coffee shops from San Francisco to New York City. Here are a few pointers for making a stellar slice right in your very own kitchen.

THE RIGHT SLICE: Start with a good-quality crusty loaf. If you buy bread that's not presliced, you get to cut it just how you like it. Littler mouths may benefit from thin slices, and bigger appetites might appreciate thick toast that's sturdy enough to handle generous toppings.

BETTER WHEN BROWNED: Toast it to your liking and serve it while still warm. The toaster isn't the only game in town when it comes to browning bread. A cast iron skillet or grill pan with a slick of olive oil adds excellent crunch as well.

BREAD LOVES BUTTER: Bread and butter are old friends for good reason: they go together deliciously. No need to go overboard here, though. A little goes a long way.

ADD A PINCH: I can't think of any type of toast—sweet or savory—that doesn't benefit from a friendly pinch of salt. It's a trick used in all the trendy toast-making cafes, because salt brightens the flavors of whatever is on the bread. If you happen to have a flaky salt, such as Maldon, this is the perfect place to use it.

8

TOAST

there was a time when I began every morning with a slice of toast, a cup of tea, and little else. It was my ritual. But I've learned that routinely starting the day like that isn't enough: I tucker out by 10 A.M. Plus, it's not exactly good role modeling: I want my kids to eat more than a skimpy slice of bread before school!

So why, then, devote an entire chapter of this book to the subject of toast? Because toast can be so much more than just a buttered slice. It can be a terrific platform for all manner of nourishing and delicious toppings. Layer on creamy cheeses, sliced vegetables, crunchy nut butter, smoked fish, fresh fruit, or toasted seeds, and it becomes something different altogether: a real breakfast, and one that takes no time at all to make.

And it's not just what's *on top of* the toast that counts, but what's *in* the toast too. Sure, you'll find French baguettes and ordinary bagels in my bread basket, but for the most part I gravitate toward whole grain loaves. These make a superior base for toast breakfasts because they're more nutrient dense and higher in fiber than white-flour bread. A hearty slice of whole grain rye bread, for example, is digested more slowly and sticks to the ribs longer than a wimpy slice of white.

What you'll find in this chapter is a "something for everyone" lineup that ranges from mega-nourishing veggie toast to a charming nut butter slice crafted to look like a teddy bear. Take your pick, or make up your own: done well, simple toast can be transformed into a very sensible meal.

makes 1 serving

"EAT YOUR VEGGIES" TARTINE

Getting kids to "eat their veggies" just got a whole lot easier with this beautiful breakfast tartine. Even a small amount of vegetables left over from dinner is worth saving, because all you'll need for topping your toast is a third of a cup. You lay prosciutto on the bread and melt cheese over the top, encasing the vegetables deliciously inside. Who can resist?

1 LARGE ¾-INCH-THICK SLICE OF CRUSTY WHOLE GRAIN BREAD, SUCH AS LEVAIN

1 THIN SLICE PROSCIUTTO

⅓ CUP LEFTOVER CHOPPED COOKED VEGETABLES, SUCH AS BELL PEPPERS, ROOT VEGETABLES, ZUCCHINI, BROCCOLI RABE, OR MUSHROOMS

ENOUGH VERY THIN SLICES OF HAVARTI OR OTHER MELTING CHEESE TO COVER THE SURFACE OF THE BREAD

1 TEASPOON BALSAMIC VINEGAR

½ TEASPOON EXTRA-VIRGIN OLIVE OIL

1. Preheat the oven or toaster oven to 425°F.
2. Place the bread on a baking sheet (small enough to fit in the toaster oven, if using). Lay the prosciutto on top of the bread. Add the vegetables and spread out in an even layer. Lay the cheese over the vegetables to cover completely.
3. Bake the bread for about 5 minutes, until the toast is crispy and the cheese melts. Remove the pan from the oven and drizzle the vinegar and oil over the toast. Cut in half and serve.

ADAPT IT: If you don't have cooked vegetables on hand, use a couple of thick slices of ripe tomato instead.

10 WAYS TO BOOST VEGGIES AT BREAKFAST

1. Zucchini—Dice and cook quickly with scrambled eggs, grate and include in breakfast muffins, or grate and stir into savory hot cereals for the last minute or two of cooking.

2. Potatoes—Grate for hash browns, or dice for breakfast hash topped with an egg.

3. Tomatoes—Tuck into breakfast sandwiches, serve beneath poached eggs, or make into fresh tomato salsa and spoon over huevos rancheros.

4. Carrots—Stir shredded carrots into muffin or pancake batter, or add to breakfast wraps.

5. Avocados—Mash onto toast, slice over fried eggs, or add to smoothies.

6. Pumpkin—Add pumpkin puree to muffins, pancakes, or smoothies.

7. Leafy greens—Blend into smoothies and green juices, add to egg dishes, or stir into savory breakfast grains.

8. Mushrooms—Sauté for scrambled eggs, or layer on top of toast with melted cheese for an open-faced sandwich.

9. Broccoli—Cook florets and add to frittatas or breakfast burritos.

10. Bell peppers—Dice and sauté with onions in scrambled eggs, or add roasted red peppers to breakfast sandwiches.

EGG AND AVOCADO SMASH

This simple recipe takes an oh-so-trendy slice of avocado toast and turns it up a notch: hard-boiled eggs add a bit of heft, and lemon juice brightens the flavors. It's a breakfast egg salad so tasty you may find yourself craving it for lunch. The mash-up of protein, healthy fats, and whole grains will satisfy even the biggest appetites in your house.

2 SLICES WHOLE GRAIN SOURDOUGH BREAD OR OTHER CRUSTY BREAD OF YOUR CHOICE

2 HARD-BOILED EGGS (SEE PAGE 53 FOR INSTRUCTIONS)

½ LARGE RIPE AVOCADO

1 ½ TEASPOONS LEMON JUICE

⅛ TEASPOON KOSHER SALT, PLUS MORE IF DESIRED

FRESHLY GROUND BLACK PEPPER

1. Toast the bread. While the bread is toasting, peel the eggs and slice them into a small bowl. Add the avocado, lemon juice, and salt. Mash the ingredients together with a fork until they form a chunky spread. Spread the egg and avocado salad evenly over the 2 slices of toast. Top with a few cracks of black pepper. Add a pinch more salt, if desired.

   BOOST IT: Lay a little pile of bean sprouts or your favorite salad greens on the toast before topping with egg salad.

·

LAYERED LOX TOAST

Open-faced lox sandwiches are a longtime breakfast favorite of mine that my kids have adopted over time. There's something irresistible about the range of flavors and textures—creamy, salty, briny, smoky, and crunchy—all on a single slice of toast. I prefer to use dense, dark German rye bread as the foundation for this, but if your crew isn't up for it, any type of sliced bread will do.

1 THIN SLICE WHOLE GRAIN RYE BREAD

1 ½ TABLESPOONS WHIPPED CREAM CHEESE

1 TEASPOON CAPERS

4 OR 5 THIN SLICES ENGLISH CUCUMBER

2 THIN SLICES LOX OR SMOKED SALMON

1 LEMON WEDGE

1. Toast the bread until crisp around the edges. (Dense, German-style rye bread will take longer to toast than other varieties.) Spread the top of the toast with the cream cheese and sprinkle with the capers. Lay the cucumber slices over the capers, followed by the lox. Squeeze a little lemon juice over the top. Cut in half and serve.

BOOST IT: If you have fresh dill on hand, chop up a bit and scatter it over the top.

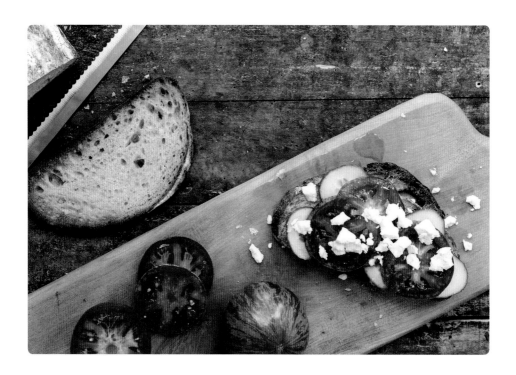

 QUICK FIX

TERRIFIC TOAST TOPPERS

Smashed avocado and
   roasted pepitas

Fresh goat cheese and sliced figs

Peanut butter, diced celery, and raisins

Cream cheese and cinnamon-sugar,
   broiled until bubbly

Hummus and grated carrots

A simple fried egg

Tahini and drizzled honey

Ricotta, sliced tomato, and chopped fresh
   basil

Warm English baked beans and shredded
   Cheddar

Almond butter and jam

Chocolate hazelnut spread and sliced
   strawberries (as a special treat)

Cream cheese, smoked salmon or smoked
   trout, and lemon juice

makes 2 slices; 1 to 2 servings

TURKISH TOAST

We took a family trip to Turkey one summer, and along with the cultural landmarks and blue seas for which the country is so famous, I fell madly in love with the breakfast they put out at our small hotel in Istanbul each morning: bread, tomatoes, cucumbers, a cheese much like feta, and olive oil. I never tired of making little open-faced sandwiches with all the fixings, and I stocked up on these ingredients as soon as I got home, just so I could continue to relish a little piece of our delicious vacation.

TWO ½-INCH-THICK SLICES OF CRUSTY WHOLE GRAIN BREAD

2 TEASPOONS EXTRA-VIRGIN OLIVE OIL

6 THIN SLICES ENGLISH CUCUMBER

4 SLICES RIPE TOMATO

SALT

⅓ CUP CRUMBLED FETA CHEESE

1. Toast the bread. Drizzle the olive oil over the top of the toast. Lay the cucumber slices over the toast, followed by the tomato slices. Add a pinch of salt and crumble the feta evenly over the top of each slice.

BOOST IT: Spread the toast with a thin layer of hummus before adding the cucumber and tomato.

makes 2 tartines; 1 to 2 servings

COTTAGE CHEESE, OLIVE OIL, AND BLACK PEPPER TARTINE

Cottage cheese may not be the prettiest ingredient in your fridge, but it is awfully handy to have around when you're in need of a quick breakfast or afternoon snack. You might be surprised by what a light drizzle of olive oil and a crack of black pepper can do for this otherwise humble slice of toast. If you aren't a fan of cottage cheese, make this with fresh ricotta instead.

ONE 5-INCH-LONG SEGMENT OF A SEEDED BAGUETTE

⅓ CUP COTTAGE CHEESE

½ TEASPOON EXTRA-VIRGIN OLIVE OIL

FRESHLY GROUND BLACK PEPPER

SALT

1. Cut the baguette in half lengthwise and lightly toast the halves. Place the toasted baguette halves cut side up. Spoon cottage cheese onto each toast and spread out evenly. Drizzle with the olive oil. Top with a crack of black pepper and a small pinch of salt.

BOOST IT: Layer paper-thin slices of radish on top of the cottage cheese to add crunch and flavor.

ADAPT IT: Skip the black pepper, and cover the top with thin slices of fresh peach or fresh berries of your choice.

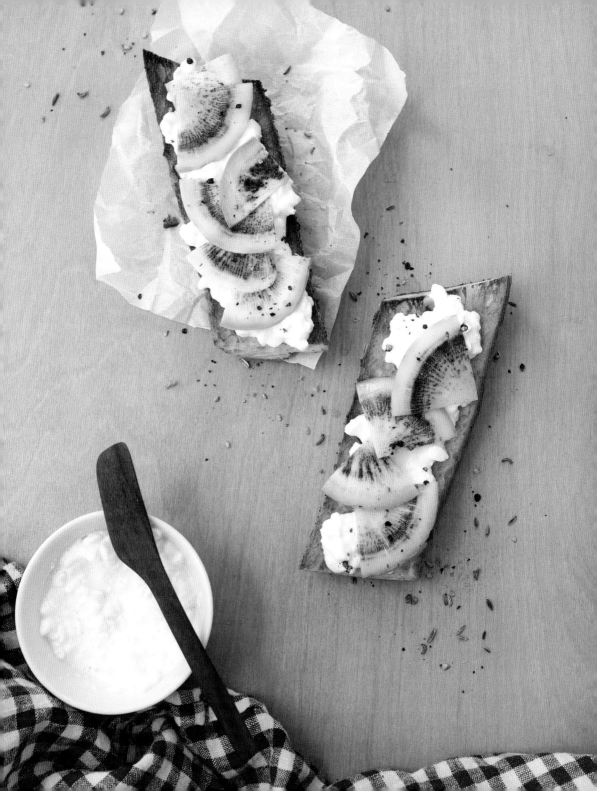

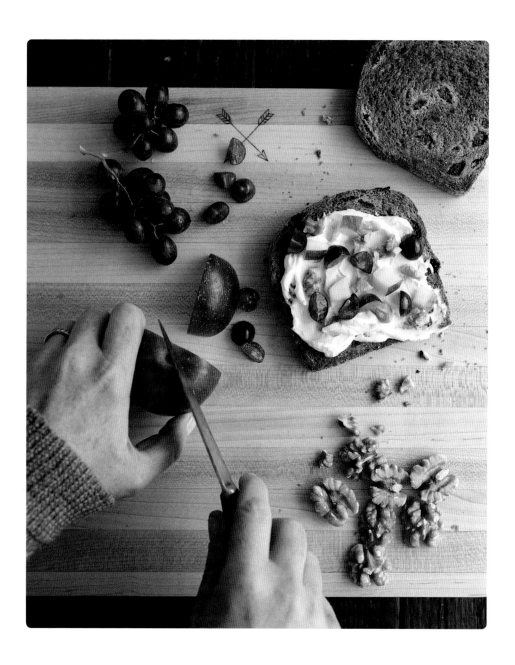

WALDORF TOAST

The Waldorf is a famous old-fashioned salad from a storied New York hotel. Who knew that the recipe would inspire a little slice of breakfast toast some hundred-plus years later? But the combination of walnuts, apples, and grapes is a good one, especially scattered over raisin toast smeared with cream cheese. Serve it at the breakfast table, or pretend you are at the Waldorf Astoria and deliver it à la room service.

1 SLICE CINNAMON-RAISIN BREAD (IDEALLY WHOLE GRAIN)

2 TABLESPOONS WHIPPED CREAM CHEESE

3 WALNUT HALVES

3 SEEDLESS GRAPES, DICED

1 TABLESPOON DICED APPLE

1. Toast the bread. Spread the top of the toast with the cream cheese. Break the walnuts into small pieces and scatter over the cream cheese, followed by the diced grapes and apple. Press lightly on the nuts and fruit to secure them on top of the cream cheese. Cut in half and serve.

TEDDY BEAR TOAST

I've never spent a whole lot of time doing "cute" when it comes to making food for my kids. That said, I'm not above pulling out the cookie cutters for sandwiches on occasion or spearing fruit onto skewers to up the fun factor. When scoring extra parenting points is as easy as toasting a slice of bread, I'm all in. Plus, this Teddy Bear number is a pretty sweet way to start your little ones off on their day.

1 SLICE WHOLE GRAIN SANDWICH BREAD

1 ½ TABLESPOONS UNSWEETENED NUT, SEED, SOY, OR PEANUT BUTTER OF YOUR CHOICE

3 THIN BANANA SLICES (ROUNDS)

3 RAISINS

1. Toast the bread and spread the nut butter evenly over the top. Place 1 banana slice in each of the top corners of the toast (for the eyes). Put the remaining banana slice in the center of the toast (for the nose). Lay a raisin on top of each banana slice.

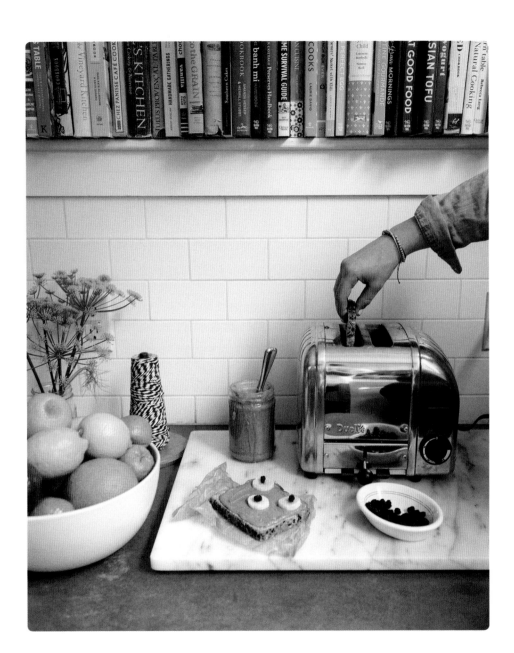

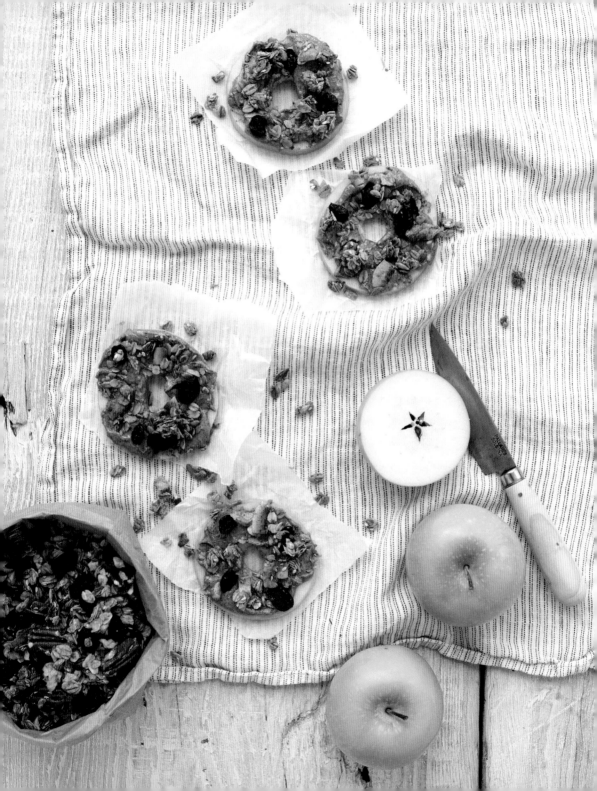

GRANOLA APPLE STACKS

I'm really stretching the notion of "toast" here by building a breakfast on top of crisp slices of apple instead of crispy slices of bread. Why not? Thin rounds of apple make a wholesome foundation for layers of nut butter and granola. Just try to eat one little slice. Impossible. They're both filling and highly addictive, in the best possible way.

1 LARGE APPLE

⅓ CUP UNSWEETENED NUT, SEED, SOY, OR PEANUT BUTTER

½ CUP GRANOLA

1. Core the apple with an apple corer or melon baller. Lay the apple on its side and cut crosswise into ¼-inch-thick slices, about 9 slices. Arrange the apple slices on a plate or work surface. Divide the nut butter evenly among the apple slices and spread it over their tops. Sprinkle the granola on top, dividing it evenly among the slices. Press the granola down lightly so it sticks to the nut butter.

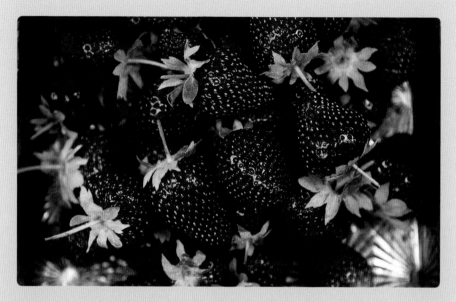

8 WAYS TO TOP A SHORT STACK

Maple syrup isn't the only ingredient in your kitchen that can top a pile of pancakes. With a little creativity, your short stack can get a whole lot more interesting and nutritious, starting with these eight topping ideas:

1. Honey Stewed Summer Fruit (see page 94)
2. Nut or seed butter
3. Sliced banana and toasted walnuts
4. Plain Greek yogurt with a spoonful of your favorite jam
5. Blueberries or blackberries heated on the stovetop, for a warm syrup
6. Applesauce and a dash of cinnamon
7. Crème fraîche and fresh berries
8. Apple butter and toasted almonds

9

PANCAKES, WAFFLES, AND FRENCH TOAST

pancakes, waffles, and french toast usually bring to mind leisurely weekend meals . . . lazy mornings spent flipping hotcakes, warming syrup, and enjoying it all while thumbing through the newspaper. But who's to say that such old favorites can't be adapted for busy weekdays too? Some folks love nothing better than to start their morning with a stack of pancakes or a crispy waffle. Why should they have to wait for the weekend?

My aim with this chapter was to tinker with traditional recipes so that they're nourishing enough for everyday eating and easy to pull off. I've relied mostly on whole grain flours, tried to work in extra protein, scaled back the sugar, and suggested ways to top a short stack with something other than heavily processed syrup. One-bowl pancakes, batters that can be mixed the night before, French toast done in the slow cooker, and a four-ingredient recipe are a few examples of what makes this chapter's offerings weekday-workable. In addition, many of the pancakes and waffles freeze well, so all you will need for getting breakfast on the table is a working toaster and a willing diner—not a particularly tall order for a very satisfying meal.

RISE AND SHINE PANCAKE MIX

I was in a pickle. The store-bought pancake mix *I* liked was deemed "too whole grainy" by my kids, but the one *they* liked didn't measure up nutritionally in my book. And so I set about making my own, a breakfast favorite. The mix comprises a combination of whole wheat, oat, and almond flour that works magic for flavor, texture, and nutritional value. You make it right in the same resealable bag (or jar) you use for storing it, which means the only cleanup is washing a few measuring cups and spoons. And, once you've got your mix done, all that you'll need to make pancakes is three ingredients and a single bowl.

PANCAKE MIX

2½ CUPS WHITE WHOLE WHEAT FLOUR OR WHOLE WHEAT PASTRY FLOUR, SPOONED AND LEVELED

1 CUP OAT FLOUR, SPOONED AND LEVELED (SEE NOTE)

1 CUP ALMOND FLOUR, SPOONED AND LEVELED (SEE NOTE)

¼ CUP DRIED BUTTERMILK (SEE PAGE 161), SPOONED AND LEVELED

3 TABLESPOONS SUGAR

1 TABLESPOON BAKING POWDER

1 TEASPOON BAKING SODA

1 TEASPOON KOSHER SALT

FOR THE PANCAKES

1 EGG

⅔ CUP WATER

2 TABLESPOONS MELTED BUTTER, PLUS MORE FOR GREASING THE PAN

1 CUP PANCAKE MIX, SPOONED AND LEVELED

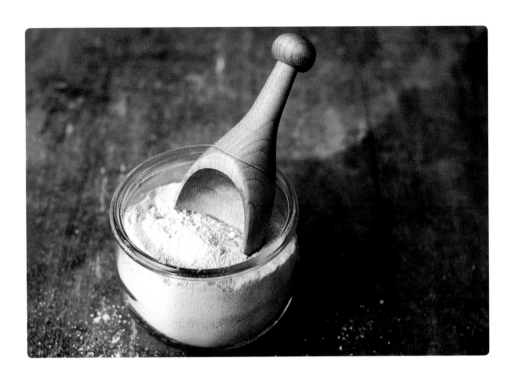

TIP | WILL THE REAL MAPLE SYRUP PLEASE STAND UP?

I grew up on "pancake syrup"—Mrs. Butterworth's, to be exact—and it took me some time to adjust to the real deal. Now, I would never go back. The difference? Mrs. Butterworth's, like most pancake syrup, contains no actual maple syrup. None. What it does have is high-fructose corn syrup and artificial flavors. Maple syrup, on the other hand, has just one ingredient—maple syrup—which comes from the sap of the sugar maple tree and is the source of several minerals. Is it more expensive than pancake syrup? Yes, but because of its natural sweetness and thin consistency, a little goes a long way. Keep in mind that although pure maple syrup is a minimally processed food, it's still in the category of sugars, so use it in moderation.

1. To make the pancake mix: Put all the Pancake Mix ingredients into a large resealable bag (or a roomy jar with a lid). Seal the bag and shake well to evenly distribute the ingredients.

2. To make the pancakes: In a medium bowl, whisk together the egg, water, and butter until combined. Add 1 cup of the Pancake Mix and stir until just incorporated. If you prefer a thicker batter, add more of the Pancake Mix, 1 tablespoon at a time. Alternatively, you can thin the batter with a little more water.

3. Set a skillet over medium heat. When the pan is hot, add a dab of butter and swirl the pan to coat the bottom. Pour some batter into the pan, figuring a little less than ¼ cup for a 4-inch pancake. Cook until bubbles appear across the surface and the bottom is golden brown. Use a spatula to flip the pancake and cook until golden brown on the second side. Transfer to a plate and serve immediately.

Note: If you don't have oat flour or almond flour, you can make your own by putting rolled oats or raw almonds into a blender and processing until it has the appearance of flour. (The almond flour will be a bit coarser than store-bought.) Be sure to measure the finished flour before adding it to the Pancake Mix.

MAKE AHEAD: The mix will keep for months if stored in a cool, dark place. The batter can be prepared the night before and stored in the refrigerator. It will thicken, so you may want to thin it with a little water in the morning before cooking.

makes about 40 silver-dollar pancakes; 3 or 4 servings

BARELY BANANA PROTEIN PANCAKES (WITH 4 LITTLE INGREDIENTS)

The batter for these protein-packed, gluten-free, pint-sized pancakes gets whirled together in one fell swoop in a blender, which doubles as the perfect pouring vessel. They are smaller and thinner than typical pancakes—think silver dollars—with a mild banana flavor that favors a swipe of tangy jam over the traditional drizzle of maple syrup. They taste best when you cook them thoroughly; they are supremely moist, so it's hard to overdo it.

3 EGGS

1 CUP OLD-FASHIONED ROLLED OATS

1 ⅓ CUPS COTTAGE CHEESE

1 SMALL RIPE BANANA

OIL OR BUTTER FOR GREASING THE SKILLET

FAVORITE JAM FOR SERVING

1. Put the eggs, oats, cottage cheese, and banana into a blender. Blend until the oats are pulverized, the cottage cheese is blended, and the batter is smooth.

2. Set a skillet over medium heat. Add about a teaspoon of oil and swirl the pan to coat the bottom. Pour about 1 tablespoon of batter into the pan for each pancake, making as many as will fit without crowding. Cook until bubbles appear across the surface and the bottom is deeply brown.

3. Use a spatula to flip the pancake and cook until firm to the touch, another 1 to 2 minutes. Serve hot out of the pan with a thin layer of jam.

BOOST IT: To make a quick blueberry syrup, cook 1½ cups fresh or frozen blueberries in a small saucepan over

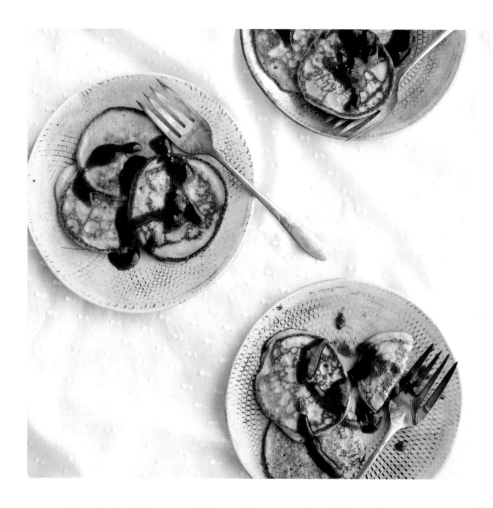

medium heat, stirring regularly, until they give off their juices and are warmed through. Add 1 tablespoon of maple syrup, stir, and serve with the pancakes.

MAKE AHEAD: These pancakes are best the morning you make them, but if you have leftover batter, store it in the fridge for the next day. The batter will be quite thick, so you'll need the aid of a spoon to spread it in the pan. Alternatively, you can thin the batter with a splash of milk.

ONE-BOWL CHILE CHEESE CORNMEAL PANCAKES

Just out of graduate school in clinical nutrition, I didn't get myself hired in a hospital cardiology unit or a diabetes clinic. Instead, I got a job interning for cookbook author Marion Cunningham, a woman who was never shy with the shortening or sugar, ingredients I had been trained to avoid. But working with Marion and witnessing her bring a book to life was terrific experience. Her recipe for simple cornmeal pancakes was one of the more memorable dishes from that time and is the inspiration for this savory breakfast. I've adapted the recipe so it is more healthful than the original, is all mixed in one bowl, and has the added kick of green chiles. The result is a pancake that's slightly crisp on the outside, tender on the inside, and when topped with grated cheese and sour cream, won't make you miss the maple syrup one bit.

1 EGG

2 TABLESPOONS OLIVE OIL, PLUS MORE FOR GREASING THE SKILLET

1 CUP MILK

½ CUP CORNMEAL

½ CUP WHITE WHOLE WHEAT FLOUR OR WHOLE WHEAT PASTRY FLOUR, SPOONED AND LEVELED

2 TEASPOONS BAKING POWDER

HEAPING ½ TEASPOON KOSHER SALT

2½ TABLESPOONS CANNED CHOPPED GREEN CHILES, DRAINED WELL

½ CUP FINELY GRATED MONTEREY JACK OR CHEDDAR CHEESE

SOUR CREAM, FOR SERVING (OPTIONAL)

1. In a medium bowl, whisk together the egg, olive oil, and milk. Add the cornmeal and flour and sprinkle the baking powder and salt over the top. Use a

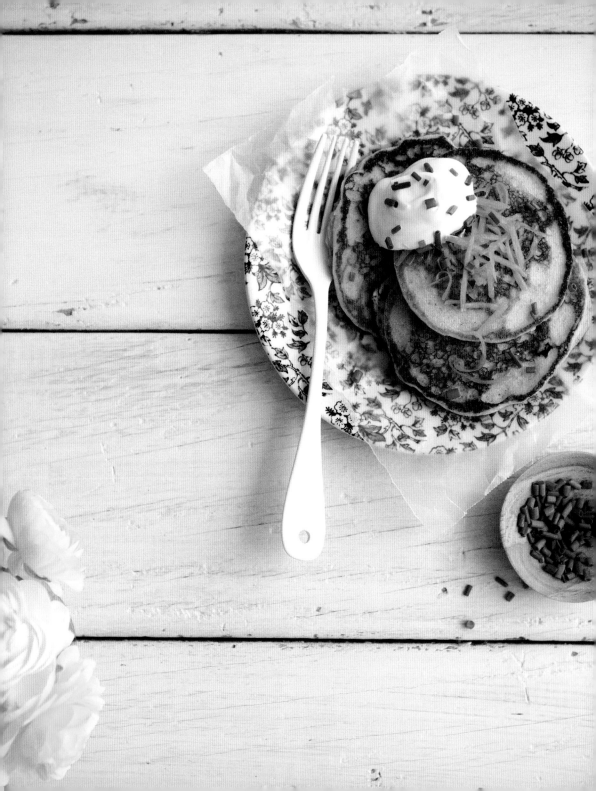

whisk to combine the ingredients until no streaks of flour and few lumps remain. Add the chiles and stir again until just mixed through. The batter will be thin, but it will puff up when cooked.

2. Set a skillet over medium heat and add a light drizzle of olive oil, swirling the pan to coat the bottom. Pour some batter into the pan, figuring ⅛ cup for a 4-inch pancake. Cook until air bubbles appear across the surface and the bottom is brown and crispy. Use a spatula to flip the pancake over and cook until brown on the second side. Transfer to a plate and add a pinch of cheese to the top, along with a dab of sour cream, if using. Eat with a knife and fork, or fold up and eat "taco style."

BOOST IT: One tablespoon of finely chopped fresh chives is a tasty addition to the batter. You can also skip the cheese and sour cream, and instead spread with cream cheese and top with cucumber slices and smoked salmon.

MAKE AHEAD: This batter can be stored overnight in the fridge. Stir it before cooking and add a little milk to thin, if needed. Once cooked, leftover pancakes can be wrapped and refrigerated. Reheat in the toaster until crispy.

QUICK FIX | **TOASTER WAFFLES THAT MAKE THE GRADE**

Nothing beats homemade waffles for taste and texture, but if you don't have time to make your own, frozen ones aren't a bad bet, as long as you choose wisely. Use a similar set of standards as when buying bread: whole grains, nothing artificial, more fiber, less sugar. Here are five that make the grade:

365 Everyday Value Organic Multigrain Waffles (Whole Foods Market brand)
Kashi 7 Grain Waffles
Nature's Path Ancient Grains Frozen Waffles
Van's 8 Whole Grains Waffles—Multigrain
Van's Gluten-Free Waffles—Ancient Grain Original

MAKE-AND-FREEZE BUTTERMILK WAFFLES

My friend Kate is an excellent person to invite over for a meal. Although she has little interest in helping at the stove, she's a champion dishwasher. The one specialty she does have are some seriously killer waffles, a recipe passed down by her grandmother. Kate's family recipe was the springboard for this one, which is a simplified version enriched with whole grain flour and flaxseed meal. They're light and crispy hot out of the pan but just as good reheated in the toaster after a time in the freezer. The only downside? They just may ruin you for store-bought frozen waffles.

1⅓ CUPS WHITE WHOLE WHEAT FLOUR OR WHOLE WHEAT FLOUR, SPOONED AND LEVELED

⅔ CUP ALL-PURPOSE FLOUR, SPOONED AND LEVELED

¼ CUP FLAXSEED MEAL, WHEAT BRAN, OR WHEAT GERM

2 TABLESPOONS PACKED BROWN SUGAR

2 TEASPOONS BAKING POWDER

½ TEASPOON BAKING SODA

1 TEASPOON KOSHER SALT

2 EGGS

2 CUPS BUTTERMILK

¼ CUP CANOLA OIL OR GRAPE SEED OIL

2 TEASPOONS VANILLA EXTRACT

1. In a large bowl, whisk together the white whole wheat flour, all-purpose flour, flaxseed meal, brown sugar, baking powder, baking soda, and salt. Set aside.

2. In a medium bowl, whisk the eggs vigorously until incorporated and bubbly. Add the buttermilk, canola oil, and vanilla. Whisk until combined and bubbly.

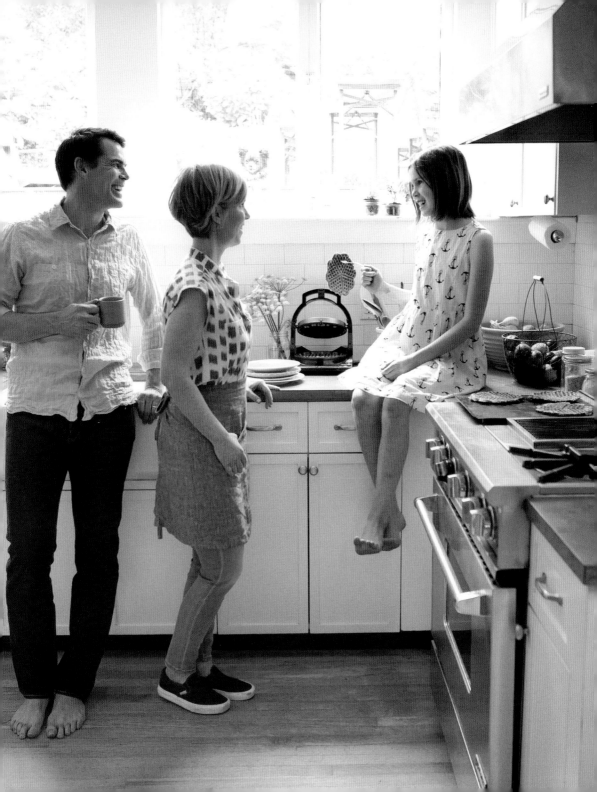

3. Pour the buttermilk mixture over the flour mixture and whisk just until smooth with few lumps remaining.

4. Preheat the waffle iron and coat it with oil or nonstick cooking spray. Pour some batter onto the waffle iron (adjust the amount based on the size of your waffle iron). Cook until the waffle is deeply golden brown and crisp. Serve immediately, or if you want everyone to eat at once, keep waffles warm in a 200°F oven until you finish cooking all the batter.

BOOST IT: The traditional method for making waffles involves separating the yolks and whites of the eggs, then beating the whites into stiff peaks and folding them into the batter at the very end. I've skipped this step in the interest of time. However, if you are making these over the weekend or have the rare luxury of time one weekday morning, feel free to whip the whites. You will find it makes the waffles especially airy.

MAKE AHEAD: This waffle batter can be made the night before and stored in the fridge. Pull it out just before you need it in the morning and stir. Once cooked and cooled, waffles can be stored in a freezer bag with the air pressed out. Reheat in the toaster.

PUMPKIN WAFFLES

Add up to ¾ cup of unsweetened pumpkin puree and 2 teaspoons of pumpkin pie spice to your waffle batter. The pumpkin and spices add great flavor, not to mention a generous amount of vitamin A and other key nutrients.

makes 2 waffle sandwiches; 2 to 4 servings

STRAWBERRY WAFFLE SANDWICH

I don't always have the time or inclination to make my own waffles. Luckily, a number of store-bought options aren't a bad bet. Sure, they'll never be as good as homemade, but when dressed up with a creamy spread and fresh berries, they make a pretty scrumptious start to the day. These sandwiches are a messy affair, so feel free to use a fork and knife if you are so inclined.

**4 WHOLE GRAIN TOASTER WAFFLES
(SEE PAGE 149 FOR SUGGESTED BRANDS; SEE ALSO BOOST IT BELOW)**

1 ½ TABLESPOONS WHIPPED CREAM CHEESE

½ CUP PLAIN GREEK YOGURT

1 TABLESPOON PURE MAPLE SYRUP

¼ TEASPOON VANILLA EXTRACT

4 MEDIUM STRAWBERRIES, SLICED

1. Toast the waffles until crisp. While the waffles are toasting, in a small bowl, vigorously whisk together the cream cheese, Greek yogurt, maple syrup, and vanilla until smooth (it's OK if tiny lumps remain).

2. Spread the cream cheese mixture evenly over 2 of the toasted waffles. Lay the sliced strawberries over the cream cheese. Cover with the remaining 2 toasted waffles. Cut each sandwich in half.

BOOST IT: Use Make-and-Freeze Buttermilk Waffles (see page 150) instead of store bought. You may need to increase the other ingredients because the waffles will be larger.

MAKE AHEAD: Make the cream cheese filling the night before, cover, and store in the refrigerator.

WEEKDAY WAFFLE IRON FRENCH TOAST

Why cook French toast in a waffle iron, you ask? Plenty of reasons: (1) While your breakfast sizzles, there's no need to keep watch. Just sit back and drink your coffee until the waffle iron beeps. (2) A waffle iron is easier and safer for kids to use on their own than a skillet over an open flame. (3) It's efficient: the top and bottom get crispy at once—no flipping required.

3 EGGS

⅔ CUP MILK

¼ CUP FRESH ORANGE JUICE (ABOUT ½ OF A JUICY ORANGE)

2 TEASPOONS VANILLA EXTRACT

5 OR 6 SLICES SOFT, SANDWICH-SIZE BREAD, SUCH AS CHALLAH OR EGG BREAD

1. Preheat the waffle iron.
2. While the waffle iron heats up, make the egg batter. In a shallow cake pan or pie tin, use a fork to whisk together the eggs, milk, orange juice, and vanilla until incorporated and a little frothy.
3. Soak a slice of bread in the batter for 15 to 30 seconds on each side, until it feels like a wet sponge.
4. Coat the waffle iron with oil or non-stick cooking spray and set the soaked bread into the waffle iron. Close the lid and cook until deeply brown and crisp. Transfer the French toast to a plate and serve with maple syrup or other favorite toppings.

BOOST IT: Add 1 to 2 teaspoons of ground cinnamon and/or 1 to 2 teaspoons of grated orange zest to bump up the flavor.

MAKE AHEAD: Store leftover French toast in a resealable bag in the fridge for up to 3 days. Reheat in a toaster.

HOW TO DRESS UP THE LEFTOVERS

When you have extra pancakes, waffles, or French toast on hand, store them for the next day and then give them a morning makeover.

- Smear cream cheese and jam between two pancakes for an easy breakfast sandwich.
- Cut waffles into bite-size pieces and thread onto skewers with strawberries in between for colorful kabobs.
- Smear nut butter and drizzle honey over thin pancakes and roll them up.
- Use cookie cutters to make charming shapes out of crispy waffles.
- Set up a pancake sundae bar with Greek yogurt, fruit, and toasted nuts or seeds.
- Cut French toast into "fingers" and serve with a little dish of warm syrup for dipping.
- Spear silver-dollar pancakes and thick banana slices with skewers.

SLOW COOKER CINNAMON FRENCH TOAST

I got the idea for doing French toast in the slow cooker from my friends Jane and Meg, the brains behind the blog *The Zen of Slow Cooking.* It's a perfect recipe to pull out when you have bits and bobs of leftover bread that need to find a home. Unless you're up at the crack of dawn, though, make it a day ahead to stow in the fridge. The kids can spoon it onto plates in the morning and warm it in the microwave. A generous spoonful of Greek yogurt and a drizzle of maple syrup are the perfect finishing touches.

1 LOAF OF CRUSTY BREAD (SUCH AS LEVAIN OR BATARD, PREFERABLY WHOLE GRAIN)

⅓ CUP GOLDEN RAISINS

4 EGGS

2 CUPS MILK

¼ CUP PURE MAPLE SYRUP

1 TEASPOON VANILLA EXTRACT

1 TEASPOON GROUND CINNAMON

GREEK YOGURT, FRESH FRUIT, AND / OR MAPLE SYRUP, FOR SERVING

1. Generously grease the inside of your slow cooker with oil.
2. Cut the bread into 1-inch cubes, enough to make 5 cups, gently packed. Store leftover bread for another use. Put the cubed bread into the slow cooker. Sprinkle the raisins over the top.
3. In a medium bowl, whisk together the eggs, milk, maple syrup, vanilla, and cinnamon until smooth.
4. Pour the egg mixture over the bread cubes. Using a fork, press down firmly on the bread cubes to soak them in the liquid a bit. The bread will bob back to the surface.

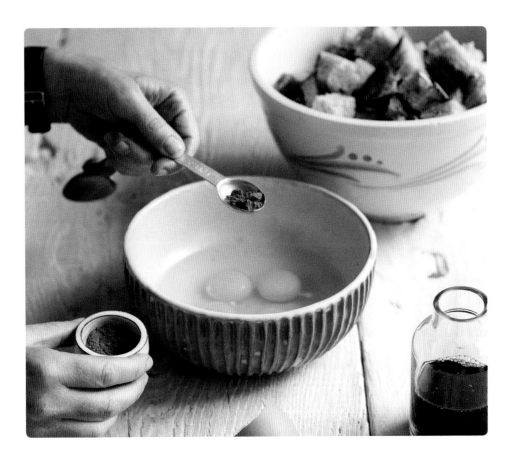

5. Secure the lid and dial the slow cooker to the high-heat setting. Cook for 2 to 2½ hours, until the egg is firm on the top and the bread is lightly crusty around the edges. Serve with yogurt, fruit, and/or maple syrup.

BOOST IT: Add ⅓ cup chopped hazelnuts or other favorite nuts when you add the raisins.

MAKE AHEAD: This can be made ahead of time, covered, and stored in the refrigerator, where it will keep for up to 3 days. To serve, spoon individual servings onto plates and reheat in the microwave.

PANCAKES, WAFFLES, AND FRENCH TOAST

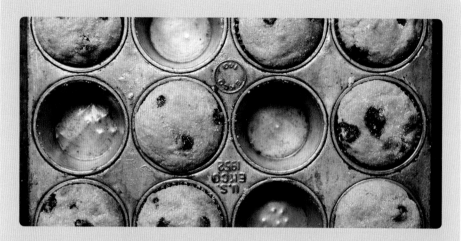

MAKE THE FREEZER YOUR FRIEND

Anytime I spy a few muffins or a couple of spare slices of quick bread that I know we might not get to before they head south, I pop them in the freezer, where they keep remarkably well. I routinely make double batches of baked goods so that I can freeze half as soon as they've cooled from the oven. I'm never sorry, particularly on days when the pantry is bare and I need breakfast for the kids, and quick. Nearly all the baked goods in this chapter freeze well for up to six weeks and defrost with relative speed. Here are a few tips for making good use of your freezer.

BREADS AND MUFFINS: Cool completely and wrap a layer of plastic wrap. Then slip bread or muffins into a resealable freezer bag with the air pressed out.

BARS: Once cool, store in a freezer bag with the air pressed out. You can also wrap each one individually in parchment paper with the ends twisted like a piece of candy before placing into the bag. That way, the kids can grab a bar right from the freezer and take it to go.

10

MAKE-AHEAD MUFFINS, BREADS, AND BARS

nothing can imitate the magic that happens when you have taken the time to stir together a batter, pour it into a loaf pan, and blast it with the heat of an oven. The aroma alone is worth the effort. That said, getting up at dawn to bake bread is not part of my routine, and I hardly expect it to be part of yours either. These are recipes you can do in advance—in the evening when the kids are tucked in or on a Saturday morning when you have a little more time. Better yet, carve out an afternoon to bake and freeze a month's worth of breakfast goodies. Invite your kids to pitch in. To me, baking is the gateway drug to cooking, and what better way to get them started than by making everyone breakfast?

This chapter is particularly well suited to the folks who don't have the time, appetite, or inclination to sit down to a meal, because every bread, muffin, and bar is perfectly portable. Pack a slice of whole grain banana bread to go, and your child can eat it on her walk to school. Or take a breakfast bar to work, saving you a trip to the coffee shop for something inferior in both taste and nutrition.

I tried to keep the recipes relatively uncomplicated. I run a home kitchen, not a pastry shop. That said, the lists of ingredients may appear long. That's because I did my best to fill every one with loads of wholesome goodies, leaning less on refined sugar than traditional recipes, while keeping the portion sizes reasonable. My hope, particularly where the kids are concerned, is that you can pair all these "make-aheads" with a glass of milk, a shmear of nut butter, or some other protein-rich side.

LEMON BLUEBERRY POLENTA MUFFINS

If you're a fan of corn muffins, this recipe might be right up your alley. It's an alternative to traditional blueberry muffins, which often have so much sugar they could pass for cupcakes. Tasty? Sure, but perhaps not the best way to start the day. Because blueberries are naturally sweet, I've found a little sugar goes a long way (each muffin has about a teaspoon). The muffins have a light lemony flavor and no shortage of juicy berries, all packaged up in a whole grain batter. Eat them for breakfast or pack them into lunch boxes. They travel well and give you something to look forward to when you reach your destination.

⅔ CUP POLENTA OR MEDIUM-GRIND CORNMEAL

1 ⅓ CUPS WHOLE WHEAT PASTRY FLOUR OR WHITE WHOLE WHEAT FLOUR, SPOONED AND LEVELED

¼ CUP PLUS 1 TABLESPOON SUGAR, DIVIDED

ZEST OF 1 LARGE LEMON

2 TEASPOONS BAKING POWDER

1 TEASPOON BAKING SODA

½ TEASPOON KOSHER SALT

2 EGGS

⅓ CUP CANOLA OIL OR GRAPE SEED OIL

1 ⅓ CUPS BUTTERMILK

1 CUP FRESH OR FROZEN BLUEBERRIES (NO NEED TO DEFROST)

1. Preheat the oven to 350°F. Generously grease 14 muffins cups with oil or nonstick cooking spray or line with paper liners.

2. In a large bowl, whisk together the polenta, whole wheat pastry flour, ¼ cup of the sugar, lemon zest, baking powder, baking soda, and salt.

3. In a medium bowl, whisk together the eggs, oil, and buttermilk until combined and smooth.

4. Pour the buttermilk mixture over the flour mixture and stir with a rubber spatula until just incorporated with no streaks of flour remaining. Add the blueberries and stir to combine.

5. Fill the prepared muffins cups nearly to the top. Sprinkle the remaining 1 tablespoon of sugar over the top of the muffins.

6. Bake for 18 to 20 minutes, until just firm to the touch on top and a toothpick inserted in the center comes out clean.

7. Let cool for a few minutes in the pan, then run a knife around the edge of each muffin and carefully wedge it out of the pan. Allow to finish cooling on the countertop.

TIP | **GOT BUTTERMILK?**

Fresh buttermilk is one ingredient I never seem to have when I need it. Luckily, fresh isn't the only way to go.

DRIED BUTTERMILK: Like its liquid counterpart, dried buttermilk lends signature tang to dressings and dips and works magic in pancakes and quick breads. Bob's Red Mill and Saco are two common brands that you will find in the baking section of many supermarkets and specialty stores, and online.

FROZEN BUTTERMILK: When you do buy fresh buttermilk, you can pack leftovers in a resealable bag or container to store in the freezer. Defrost it in the fridge before using.

BUTTERMILK SUBSTITUTE: You can make a buttermilk "stand-in" that does the job of real buttermilk, though it falls a bit short on flavor. Here's the formula: In place of 1 cup of buttermilk, mix 1 tablespoon lemon juice or white vinegar into 1 cup minus 1 tablespoon of milk. Allow it to sit at room temperature for 5 minutes, stir, and then use as needed.

DOUBLE PUMPKIN PIE MUFFINS

Pumpkin isn't just for Halloween or Thanksgiving. Both the flesh and seeds are nutrient rich and available year-round on supermarket shelves. Take full advantage of both of these healthy "convenience foods" by baking tender, tasty breakfast muffins, each of which delivers 40 percent of your daily need for vitamin A and a respectable amount of protein and iron, all at about 200 calories (far less than the typical store-bought muffin). Best of all, they're bakeshop beautiful and just as scrumptious.

¾ CUP RAW PEPITAS (SHELLED PUMPKIN SEEDS)

1 ⅓ CUPS WHOLE WHEAT PASTRY FLOUR OR WHITE WHOLE WHEAT FLOUR, SPOONED AND LEVELED

¼ CUP PACKED BROWN SUGAR

1 ½ TEASPOONS BAKING SODA

1 TEASPOON BAKING POWDER

1 TABLESPOON PUMPKIN PIE SPICE (OR 1 ½ TEASPOONS GROUND CINNAMON,
1 TEASPOON GROUND GINGER, ¼ TEASPOON GROUND NUTMEG, AND ¼ TEASPOON GROUND CLOVES)

½ TEASPOON KOSHER SALT

1 EGG

¾ CUP PUMPKIN PUREE (NOT PUMPKIN PIE FILLING)

¼ CUP MILK

½ CUP HONEY

⅓ CUP CANOLA OIL OR GRAPE SEED OIL

1. Preheat the oven to 350°F. Grease 15 muffin cups with oil or nonstick cooking spray or line with paper liners.

2. Put the pepitas into a blender and run until they're the texture of flour, being careful not to overdo it (or you'll make

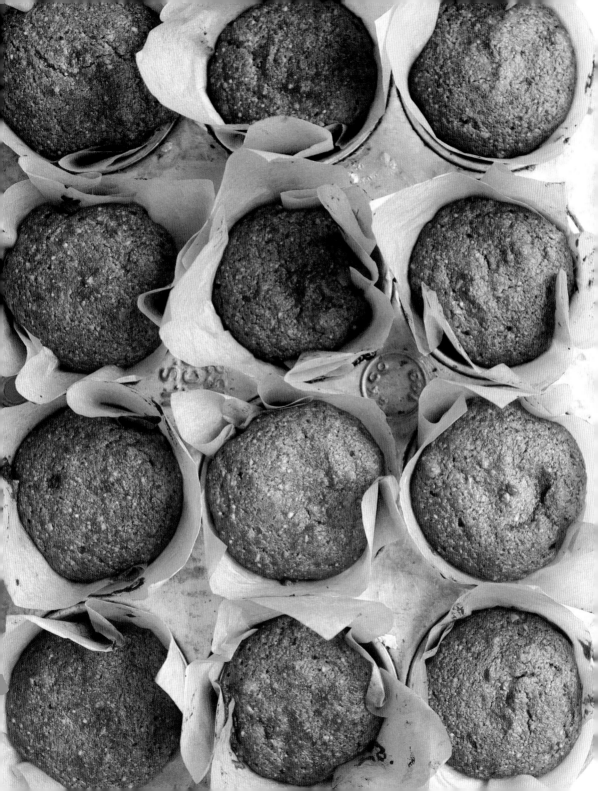

pumpkin seed butter). Transfer to a large bowl and add the whole wheat pastry flour, brown sugar, baking soda, baking powder, pumpkin pie spice, and salt. Whisk well to combine.

3. In a medium bowl, whisk together the egg, pumpkin puree, milk, honey, and oil until smooth and combined. Pour over the flour mixture and stir with a rubber spatula just until smooth with no streaks of flour remaining.

4. Pour the batter into the prepared muffin cups, filling them to ¼-inch shy of the top.

5. Bake for about 20 minutes, until just firm to the touch and a toothpick inserted in the center comes out clean.

6. Let cool for a few minutes in the pan, then run a knife around the edge of each muffin and wedge it out of the pan. They are delicate, so be gentle. Allow to finish cooling on the countertop.

BOOST IT: "Frost" the muffins with whipped cream cheese.

MAKE AHEAD: Make the wet mixture and the dry mixture the night before. Cover the wet mixture and store in the fridge. In the morning, preheat the oven, combine the mixtures, and fill the muffin cups. When you bake the muffins, add 1 or 2 extra minutes of baking time because the ingredients will be cold.

WHAT TO DO WITH THAT EXTRA PUMPKIN

Open a can of pumpkin for a batch of muffins, and you're likely to have a little left over. Even a small amount is nutrient rich and flavor packed, so don't banish it to the compost. Here are a few ideas for using up every last bite:

- Stir a spoonful into your morning oatmeal along with a dash of cinnamon.
- Make a creamy pumpkin smoothie. A quick Internet search will turn up plenty of recipes.
- Add it to your waffle batter (pages 150–152).
- Pack leftovers into a container and freeze for the next time you want to make muffins.

GOOD MORNING SUNSHINE MUFFINS

Waking up to a dozen of these moist and tender muffins makes for a good morning indeed. You'll find about three and a half cups of fruits, vegetables, and nuts in every batch, which means there's no shortage of texture and flavor. It's a throwback to the morning glory muffin from the '70s, only made with pear instead of apple, whole grain flour instead of white, and a lot less sugar and oil than the original. Enlist the help of a food processor to quickly grate the pear and carrots, and you will cut down on prep time too.

2 EGGS

¼ CUP MILK

½ CUP EXTRA-VIRGIN OLIVE OIL

¼ CUP PURE MAPLE SYRUP

1 LARGE SLIGHTLY RIPE PEAR, SUCH AS D'ANJOU OR BARTLETT, COARSELY GRATED

2 MEDIUM CARROTS, COARSELY GRATED

½ CUP CHOPPED PECANS OR WALNUTS

½ CUP UNSWEETENED SHREDDED COCONUT

⅓ CUP RAISINS

1 ½ CUPS WHOLE WHEAT PASTRY FLOUR OR WHITE WHOLE WHEAT FLOUR, SPOONED AND LEVELED

¼ CUP PACKED BROWN SUGAR

1 ½ TEASPOONS BAKING SODA

1 ½ TEASPOONS GROUND CINNAMON

¾ TEASPOON GROUND GINGER

½ TEASPOON KOSHER SALT

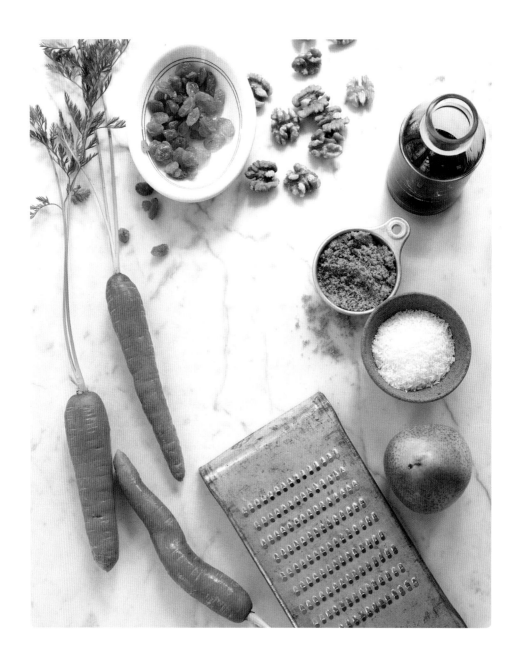

1. Preheat the oven to 350°F. Grease 12 muffin cups with oil or nonstick cooking spray or line with paper liners.

2. Whisk the eggs in a large bowl until incorporated. Add the milk, olive oil, and maple syrup and whisk until combined. Add the pear (with its juices), carrots, pecans, coconut, and raisins and stir until the ingredients are evenly distributed in the liquid.

3. In a medium bowl, whisk together the whole wheat pastry flour, brown sugar, baking soda, cinnamon, ginger, and salt until combined. Add to the wet mixture and stir with a rubber spatula just until no streaks of flour remain and the ingredients are combined.

4. Spoon the batter into the prepared muffin cups nearly to the top.

5. Bake for about 20 minutes, until a toothpick inserted into the center comes out clean.

6. Let cool for a few minutes in the pan, then run a knife around the edge of each muffin and carefully wedge it out of the pan. Allow to finish cooling on the countertop.

MAKE AHEAD: The batter can be made the night before, covered, and stored immediately in the refrigerator. In the morning, preheat the oven, fill the muffin cups, and bake. Figure an extra 1 or 2 minutes of baking time because the batter will be cold. The rise may not be quite as high as muffins made with fresh batter, but they will be warm and tasty nevertheless.

makes 1 loaf

BANANA CHOCOLATE CHIP MILLET BREAD (FOR SLOW COOKER OR OVEN)

You don't have to make this bread in a slow cooker, but it's nice to know that you can. The upside is that you don't have to stick around while the baking happens. Get it going in the slow cooker and pop out to run errands or collect kids from school. You'll come home to a supremely moist, warm loaf of banana bread. What could be better? Bake it in the oven, and the job will go about twice as fast, and the result will be a more beautifully burnished crust. Either way, you've got something wholesome for breakfast, made with whole wheat flour, crunchy millet, and just enough dark chocolate to keep the kids asking for seconds.

3 MEDIUM RIPE BANANAS

⅓ CUP CANOLA OR GRAPE SEED OIL

2 EGGS

⅓ CUP HONEY

1 TEASPOON VANILLA EXTRACT

1¾ CUP WHOLE WHEAT PASTRY FLOUR OR WHITE WHOLE WHEAT FLOUR, SPOONED AND LEVELED

¼ CUP MILLET

1 TEASPOON BAKING SODA

½ TEASPOON KOSHER SALT

⅓ CUP DARK CHOCOLATE CHIPS

1. This bread is made in a 9 × 5-inch loaf pan. Check to make sure that the pan fits inside your slow cooker before you begin. If not, bake in the oven.

2. If using a slow cooker, dial it to the high-heat setting. If using the oven, preheat it to 350°F.

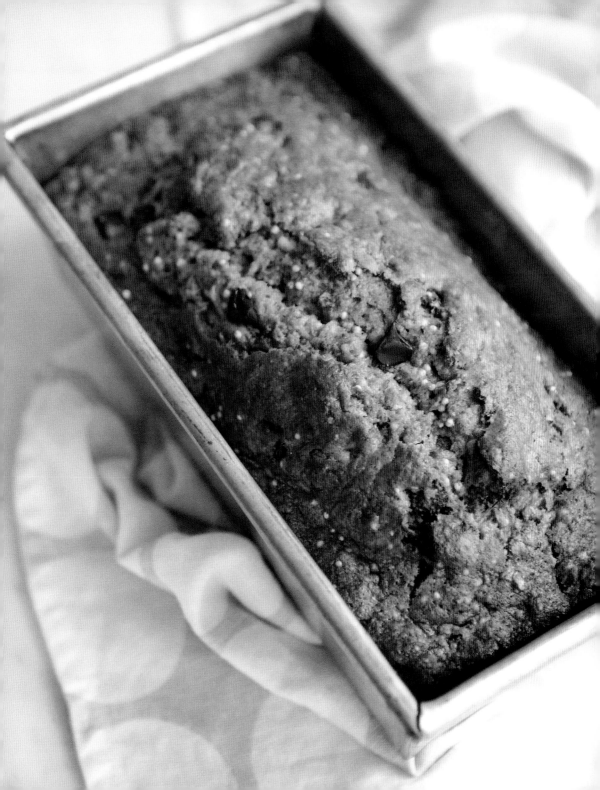

3. Generously grease a 9 × 5-inch loaf pan with oil or nonstick cooking spray.

4. Put the bananas into a large bowl and mash into a lumpy puree with a fork. Add the canola oil, eggs, honey, and vanilla. Stir with the fork until combined.

5. In a separate large bowl, stir together the whole wheat pastry flour, millet, baking soda, and salt with a fork until combined.

6. Add the flour mixture to the banana mixture and stir with a rubber spatula just until combined with no visible streaks of flour. Add the chocolate chips and stir again.

7. Pour the batter into the prepared loaf pan.

8. Set the loaf pan in the slow cooker and secure the lid, or put it into the oven. Bake until the bread is firm when pressed gently with a finger and a toothpick inserted into the center comes out clean (test in a few spots). This will take about 2¼ to 2½ hours in the slow cooker or 1 hour in the oven.

BOOST IT: Toast a slice of banana bread and spread with your favorite nut or seed butter or whipped cream cheese.

ADAPT IT: If you don't have or don't care for millet, use ⅓ cup finely chopped pecans or walnuts instead.

 QUICK FIX | A GLASS OF MORNING MILK

On those "wrong side of the bed" mornings when breakfast is of little interest, my fallback has always been, "have a glass of milk." In our house that usually means a cup of cow's milk, but soy milk will also provide protein, calcium (if fortified), and hydration. Pairing the muffins, breads, and bars in this chapter with a glass of milk rounds out the meal, providing a good boost of nutrition.

makes 1 loaf

NO-KNEAD BROWN BREAD

Many of us are a little bit terrified by the idea of making yeast breads. Myself included. You have to count on all that chemistry, to trust that the yeast and heat will react as you want them to so that your bread will indeed rise. This simple loaf, however, is easier on the baker than most. There is no kneading involved—just a handful of vigorous turns with a sturdy spoon and one relatively brief rise. The dough is mostly whole wheat, with just enough rye to add an earthy tang that reminds me of sourdough. The result is a homey, wholesome loaf that, when cut into thick slices and slathered with salted butter . . . well, there's nothing quite like it. Plus, your kitchen will smell like a bread shop.

2 CUPS WARM WATER (95°F TO 115°F)

½ TABLESPOON BLACKSTRAP MOLASSES

1 TABLESPOON ACTIVE DRY YEAST (A LITTLE MORE THAN 1 PACKET)

2 CUPS WHOLE WHEAT FLOUR (NOT WHOLE WHEAT PASTRY FLOUR), SPOONED AND LEVELED

1 CUP ALL-PURPOSE FLOUR, SPOONED AND LEVELED

¾ CUP RYE FLOUR, SPOONED AND LEVELED

1 ½ TEASPOONS KOSHER SALT

1 TABLESPOON BUTTER, MELTED

1 TABLESPOON SESAME SEEDS

SALTED BUTTER, AT ROOM TEMPERATURE, FOR SERVING

1. Preheat the oven to 425°F.
2. In a small bowl, stir together the water and molasses until the molasses dissolves. Sprinkle the yeast over the top, jiggle the bowl a bit so the water engulfs the yeast, and set in a warm place

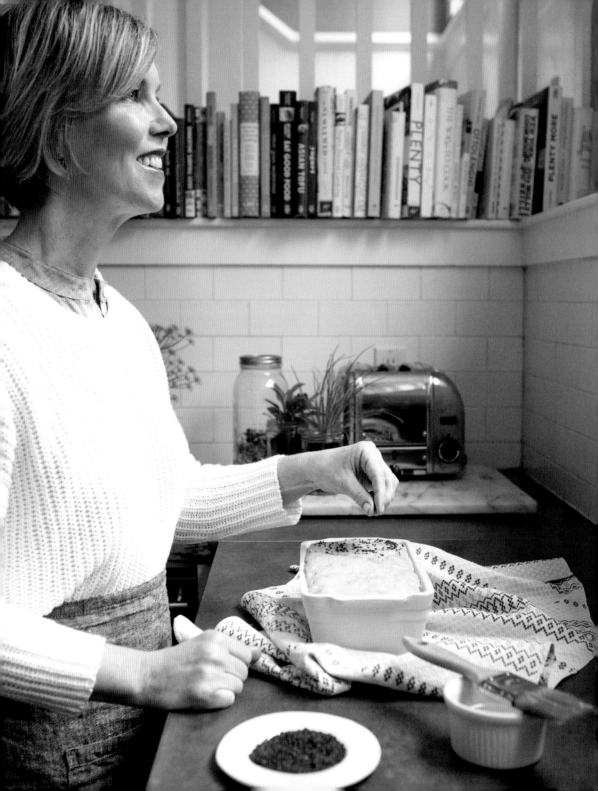

until the yeast liquefies and swells and tiny air bubbles appear, about 5 minutes.

3. In a large bowl, whisk together the whole wheat flour, all-purpose flour, rye flour, and salt. Pour the yeast and water mixture over the flour and use a sturdy spoon to stir it very thoroughly and vigorously to blend the ingredients and distribute the yeast (unlike muffin and quick bread batter, you needn't worry about overworking the dough). Cover the bowl with a damp kitchen towel and set in a warm place to rise (I set it on top of the stove).

4. When the dough has nearly doubled in size (about 30 minutes), give it several vigorous strokes with a spoon to deflate the loaf and work out the air bubbles.

5. Use a pastry brush to grease the inside of a 9 × 5-inch loaf pan with the melted butter, reserving just a little bit for the top of the bread. Transfer the dough to the pan, dab the remaining butter on top of the dough, and sprinkle it with the sesame seeds.

6. Put the loaf pan into the oven and bake for about 1 hour, until the bread is deeply brown and sounds hollow when you tap it firmly with your hand.

7. Remove the pan from the oven, run a knife around the edges of the bread, and turn it out from the pan. Set it upright and leave it to cool for at least 30 minutes before slicing. (It pays to be patient here.) Serve sliced, toasted, and spread with salted butter.

CHEESY ZUCCHINI AND OLIVE BREAD

This isn't your ordinary zucchini bread. It's savory rather than sweet—a departure from typical breakfast breads, which err in the opposite direction. Treat the dough like you do the kids on your very best day: with a gentle hand. Quick breads don't like an aggressive baker, so stir the batter enough to make the ingredients come together but no more. The payoff will be a golden loaf with a tender crumb punctuated by nuggets of cheese and salty olives. Cut it into generous slices, and get it warm and crusty in the toaster.

2 CUPS COARSELY GRATED ZUCCHINI (ABOUT 2 MEDIUM ZUCCHINI)

1 ½ TEASPOONS KOSHER SALT, DIVIDED

1 ½ CUPS WHITE WHOLE WHEAT FLOUR OR WHOLE WHEAT PASTRY FLOUR, SPOONED AND LEVELED

1 CUP ALL-PURPOSE FLOUR, SPOONED AND LEVELED

2 TEASPOONS BAKING POWDER

½ TEASPOON BAKING SODA

¼ TEASPOON FRESHLY GROUND BLACK PEPPER

2 EGGS

⅓ CUP EXTRA-VIRGIN OLIVE OIL

½ CUP PLAIN YOGURT

½ CUP MILK

3 SCALLIONS, THINLY SLICED, WHITE AND LIGHT GREEN PARTS ONLY

½ CUP PITTED KALAMATA OLIVES, ROUGHLY CHOPPED

4 OUNCES SHARP CHEDDAR CHEESE, CUT INTO ⅓-INCH CUBES (A LITTLE OVER ¾ CUP)

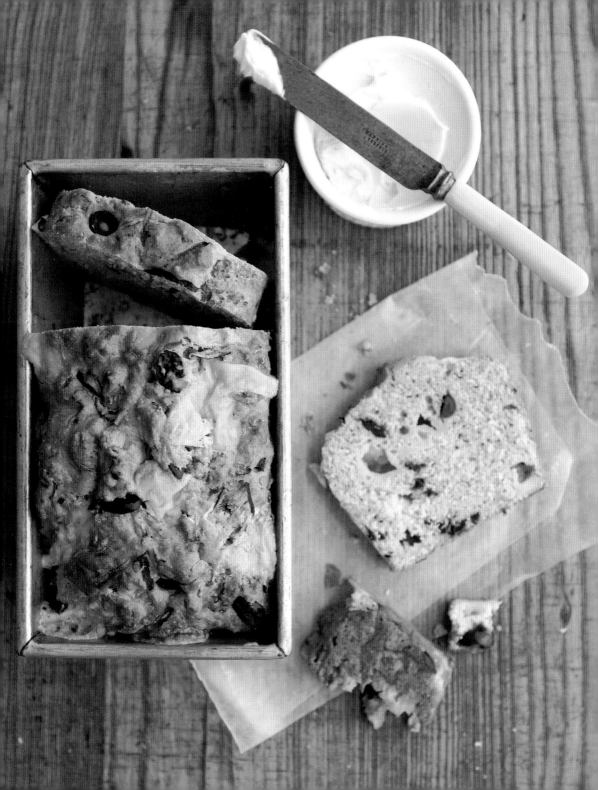

1. Preheat the oven to 350°F. Generously grease a 9 × 5-inch loaf pan with oil or nonstick cooking spray and set aside.

2. Put the zucchini into a colander set in the sink. Sprinkle with 1 teaspoon of the salt and use your hands to toss together. Leave the zucchini in the colander to allow the salt to draw out some of its liquid.

3. In a large bowl, whisk together the white whole wheat flour, all-purpose flour, baking powder, baking soda, black pepper, and the remaining ½ teaspoon of the salt.

4. In a medium bowl, whisk together the eggs, olive oil, yogurt, and milk until combined.

5. Returning to the zucchini, squeeze it thoroughly to extract excess liquid, allowing it to drain through the colander. Do this several times to eliminate as much of the moisture as possible. The zucchini will remain moist but should not be wet. Add it to the egg mixture. Add the scallions and olives and stir well with a spoon.

6. Add the egg mixture to the flour mixture and stir gently with a spoon just until the streaks of flour disappear. Add the cheese and stir just enough to distribute it throughout the dough, being careful not to overmix.

7. Transfer the dough to the prepared loaf pan and use a spoon (or your fingers) to smooth the top a bit. It will be rough and craggy.

8. Bake for about 1 hour and 10 minutes, until the loaf is golden and a toothpick inserted into the center comes out clean. If you aren't sure if it's done, remove the loaf and pat it firmly with your hand: it should sound hollow.

9. Remove from the oven and allow the bread to cool in the pan for 5 minutes. Run a knife around the edge of the bread, tip the pan over, and gently dislodge the bread onto the countertop. Set it upright and allow to cool for at least 30 minutes. Serve sliced, toasted, and spread lightly with butter.

BOOST IT: Top the toasted bread with smoked salmon.

ADAPT IT: Leave out the olives.

BIRDSEED BARS

When I first began cooking with millet, I learned that it's a common ingredient in garden-variety birdseed. I imagine birds are fond of pumpkin and chia seeds too, which is why I named these Birdseed Bars. The method for making them is pretty simple. The nuts and seeds get toasted on a single baking sheet until fragrant and then bound with a blend of dates, honey, and nut butter. After that, no further baking is required, just a tiny drizzle of dark chocolate. The result is a bang-up breakfast bar that is crunchy, chewy, and flavorful . . . a mini meal that is most definitely *not* for the birds.

1¼ CUPS OLD-FASHIONED ROLLED OATS (NOT QUICK OATS)

½ CUP SLICED ALMONDS

⅓ CUP RAW PEPITAS (SHELLED PUMPKIN SEEDS)

¼ CUP MILLET

½ CUP UNSWEETENED SHREDDED COCONUT

1 TABLESPOON CHIA SEEDS

⅓ CUP DRIED CRANBERRIES OR DRIED CHERRIES

½ TEASPOON KOSHER SALT

5 LARGE MEDJOOL DATES, PITTED

¼ CUP UNSWEETENED ALMOND BUTTER, PEANUT BUTTER, OR SUNFLOWER BUTTER

¼ CUP HONEY

2 TABLESPOONS WATER

3 TABLESPOONS BITTERSWEET CHOCOLATE CHIPS

1. Preheat the oven to 350°F. Line an 8 × 8-inch baking pan with a piece of parchment paper large enough that it drapes over two sides.

2. Put the oats, almonds, pepitas, millet, and coconut on a large baking sheet and spread out to cover the entire surface evenly. Bake for about 10 minutes, until the oats are fragrant and the coconut is browned. Remove from the oven and transfer to a large bowl. Add the chia seeds, dried cranberries, and salt and stir well.

3. Put the dates, nut butter, honey, and water into the bowl of a food processor fitted with a metal blade. Process until the ingredients incorporate to form a thick paste, stopping to scrape down the sides as needed. (Tiny flecks of date skins will remain throughout.)

4. Spoon the nut butter mixture into the bowl with the oats. Using the sides of a rubber spatula, press and stir the ingredients together until thoroughly combined. Your hands can help with this if you don't mind getting a little sticky.

5. Dump the dough into the prepared 8 × 8-inch baking pan and use your hands to press it *very firmly* into the bottom, creating an even layer that fills the entire bottom of the pan. (It will help to put an extra piece of parchment on top of the dough so your hands won't stick as you press down.)

6. Put the chocolate chips into a small microwave-safe bowl or ramekin and microwave on high in 30-second bursts, stirring after each one, until the chocolate is smooth, about 1½ minutes. Stir the chocolate again with a fork and then use the fork to drizzle it over the top of the bars (you may need to flick the fork a bit to release the chocolate). Put the pan into the freezer for 30 minutes, or until firm.

7. Remove the pan from the freezer. Run a knife around the edge of the dough and use the two draping sides of parchment to lift it out of the pan. Transfer to a cutting surface and use a large knife to cut the block into 12 bars.

8. Store bars in a resealable bag or airtight container. Keep them in the refrigerator, where they will stay nice and chewy.

MAKE AHEAD: Bars will keep in the fridge for several weeks. They can also be stored in the freezer.

MILK AND CEREAL BARS

I think of these as "desperate times" bars. They're good ones to have on hand for those mornings when the machine of getting kids up and out the door feels a little rusty and breakfast is practically an afterthought. One or two of these along with a glass of cold milk is enough to fuel a morning and is better than a store-bought cereal bar any day.

3 CUPS "O" CEREAL, SUCH AS CHEERIOS

½ CUP ROASTED SALTED PEANUTS

⅓ CUP NONFAT DRIED MILK POWDER

¼ CUP FLAXSEED MEAL

½ TEASPOON GROUND CINNAMON

½ CUP UNSWEETENED PEANUT BUTTER

¼ CUP HONEY

¼ CUP BROWN RICE SYRUP

1 TABLESPOON WATER

1. Line an 8 × 8-inch baking pan with a piece of parchment paper large enough that it drapes over two sides.
2. Put the "O" cereal, peanuts, milk powder, flaxseed meal, and cinnamon in a large bowl. Stir well and set aside.
3. Put the peanut butter, honey, rice syrup, and water in a small saucepan over medium-high heat. Cook, stirring occasionally, for about 2 to 3 minutes, until the mixture is well combined and begins to bubble around the rim. Pour the peanut butter syrup over the cereal mixture and stir immediately, while still hot, until the syrup evenly and thoroughly coats the cereal mixture.

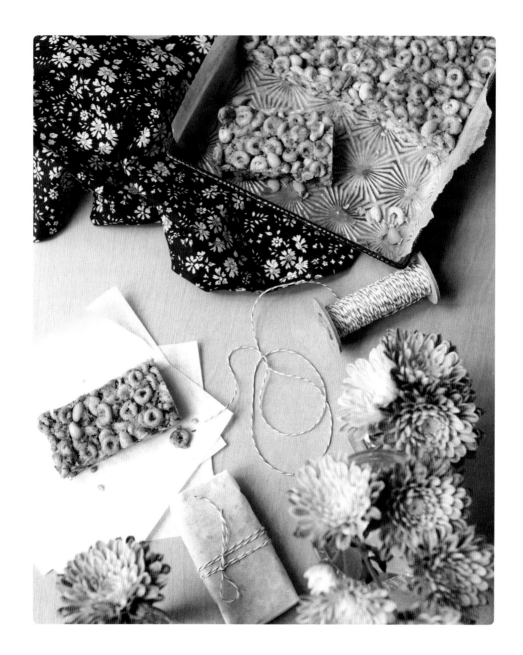

4. Dump the mixture into the prepared pan and allow to cool slightly, until just barely cool enough to touch. Grease your hands generously with oil and press the mixture *very firmly* into the bottom of the pan, creating an even layer that fills the entire bottom of the pan. (Alternatively, lay a piece of parchment over the mixture as you press down, so it doesn't stick to your hands.) Allow to cool completely.

5. Run a knife around the edge of the dough and use the two draping sides of parchment to lift it out of the pan. Transfer to a cutting surface and use a large knife to cut the block into squares.

6. Stack bars in an airtight container and store in the refrigerator for up to 1 week. The bars are sticky, so place a piece of parchment paper between layers.

BAKED APPLESAUCE MOLASSES DONUTS

I don't make these often for weekday breakfasts, but when I do, the kids are quick to show up in the kitchen. My preference is to mix the batter the night before, so all I need to do in the morning is to fill a donut pan and get it into a hot oven. Because these donuts are baked instead of fried, there's no boiling oil to contend with and the fat content is cut in half, at least. If you don't have a donut pan already, get hold of one: a single batch of these beauties is worth the ten bucks it will set back your bank account.

DONUTS

1 CUP WHOLE WHEAT PASTRY FLOUR, SPOONED AND LEVELED

¾ TEASPOON BAKING SODA

1 TEASPOON GROUND CINNAMON

¼ TEASPOON GROUND ALLSPICE

¼ TEASPOON GROUND GINGER

⅛ TEASPOON GROUND NUTMEG

¼ TEASPOON KOSHER SALT

¾ CUP UNSWEETENED APPLESAUCE

⅓ CUP PACKED BROWN SUGAR

1 ½ TABLESPOONS BLACKSTRAP MOLASSES

1 EGG

¼ CUP CANOLA OIL OR GRAPE SEED OIL

1 TEASPOON VANILLA EXTRACT

2 TABLESPOONS SUGAR

½ TEASPOON GROUND CINNAMON

2 TABLESPOONS BUTTER, MELTED

1. Put the oven rack in the middle position and preheat to 325°F. Generously grease a donut pan with oil or nonstick cooking spray. (Start by greasing 9 wells, then grease more if needed—the number of donuts will vary depending on the size of your pans.)

2. In a large bowl, whisk together the flour, baking soda, cinnamon, allspice, ginger, nutmeg, and salt.

3. In a medium bowl, whisk together the applesauce, brown sugar, molasses, egg, canola oil, and vanilla until well combined.

4. Add the applesauce mixture to the flour mixture and whisk just until smooth.

5. Transfer the batter to a glass measuring cup with a lip for pouring or a small pitcher and fill each donut well to about ¼-inch shy of the top.

6. Bake for 13 to 15 minutes, until the top of a donut springs back when lightly pressed and a toothpick inserted in the center comes out clean. The cooking time may vary depending on the size of your pans. Remove the pans from the oven and allow to cool on the countertop for 5 minutes. Invert the pans to gently release the donuts.

7. To top the warm donuts, combine the sugar and cinnamon in a bowl just large enough to accommodate 1 donut. Use a pastry brush to lightly coat the top of a donut with butter, then immediately invert the donut into the cinnamon sugar, rolling it around so the top and sides are lightly coated. Set aside and continue to top the remaining donuts.

8. These donuts are best eaten warm from the oven, but they will taste good for up to 3 days. Store in an airtight container.

MAKE AHEAD: The batter can be made a day ahead, covered, and stored immediately in the refrigerator. In the morning, pull it out and leave it on the counter to warm up a bit while the oven heats.

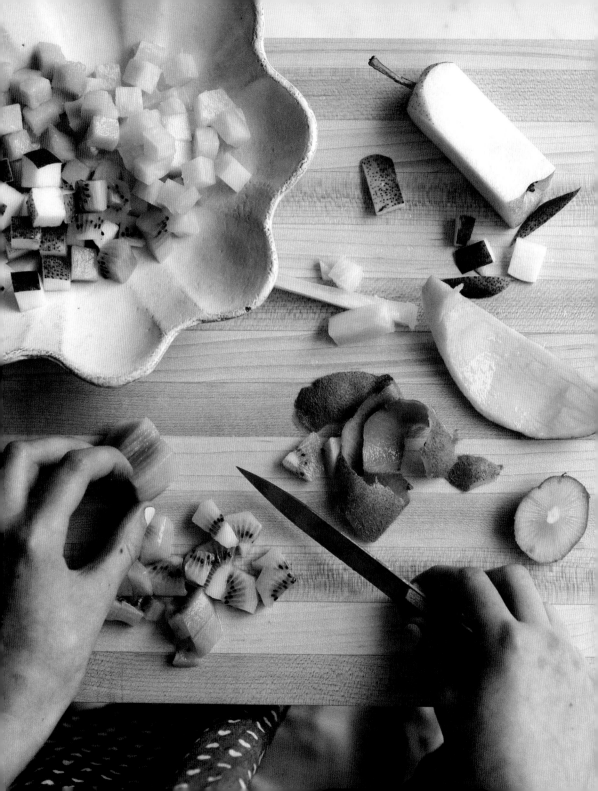

11
WEEKEND FAVORITES

there's no doubt that once kids come onto the scene, our weekends never quite recover. Sleeping in becomes a thing of the past, and uninterrupted time with the Sunday paper? A distant memory. But occasionally, maybe—barring soccer games and swim meets—we can carve out a little more room for breakfast than weekday mornings afford.

In our house, we don't do brunch every weekend, but I relish those mornings when we do manage to pull something together. I'll get a batch of crepes going, and everyone will try their hand with the buckwheat batter. Or my husband will cook up a big pan of his famous huevos rancheros, which never disappoint.

One of my favorite ways to spend a weekend morning is with an early trip to the farmers' market followed by brunch using the spoils of my shopping. We set a proper table, and we eat out in our little urban backyard if the sun is shining. We linger.

In this chapter, I've pulled together our family's weekend favorites, the ones we've made time and again, along with a few that are new to our table. I've included a broad range—from sweet to savory, from simple to sophisticated, from wholesome to a little more indulgent. My kids are crazy about the Blackberry Orange Puffy Pancake (page 188), I'm mad for Grapefruit Brûlée (page 186), and my husband is a hash guy, so that root vegetable number (Roasted Root Hash with Poached Eggs, page 199) is for him.

Take the time, gather your people, and make a real breakfast this weekend.

GRAPEFRUIT BRÛLÉE WITH MINT AND CRÈME FRAÎCHE

Several years ago, my mother-in-law gave me a mini blowtorch for Christmas. Beyond making the occasional crème brûlée, it didn't get much play in the kitchen. But then I discovered that by sprinkling sugar over a halved grapefruit and applying a bit of heat, I could achieve a deliciously crackled top on that too. The kids were smitten, and we've been making it ever since. Luckily, there's no need for a blowtorch here—your oven's broiler will do. All on its own, the brûléed grapefruit is delicious, but with the addition of crème fraîche and mint? Transformative.

2 LARGE GRAPEFRUITS (IDEALLY RED GRAPEFRUITS BECAUSE THEY'RE SO PRETTY)

2 TABLESPOONS BROWN SUGAR (NOT PACKED)

4 MINT LEAVES, CUT INTO CHIFFONADE OR ROUGHLY CHOPPED

2 TABLESPOONS CRÈME FRAÎCHE

1. Put the oven rack in the highest position and turn on the broiler.
2. Cut the grapefruits in half crosswise (not through the stem end). For each half, run a sharp paring knife around the perimeter of the skin to separate the main flesh from the peel, then cut along the membranes to free each triangle segment of fruit so that it's easy to dislodge with a spoon.
3. Put the grapefruit halves on a baking sheet, cut side up. Blot the juices off the top of each with a paper towel to dry. Sprinkle the brown sugar over the tops and set the baking sheet into the oven under the broiler. Broil 30 to 60 seconds, until the sugar melts and bubbles.
4. Remove the pan from the oven and transfer the grapefruit halves to a serving platter. Scatter the mint over the top. Spoon the crème fraîche into a ramekin or small bowl to serve on the side. Serve immediately.

A LITTLE FRUIT SALAD

It's the little things, sometimes, that make all the difference in a recipe. Take this salad, for instance, which isn't exactly groundbreaking. It's fruit salad, after all, with a splash of vanilla. But because it features five different fruits cut into tiny pieces, you get loads of flavor in every mouthful. Plus, the orange, yellows, and greens make for a pretty bowl. It's one I find kids especially love.

⅓ OF A FRESH PINEAPPLE, CUT INTO ⅓-INCH DICE (ABOUT 1 HEAPING CUP)

1 LARGE RIPE MANGO, CUT INTO ⅓-INCH DICE

4 MEDIUM KIWIFRUITS, PEELED AND CUT INTO ⅓-INCH DICE

1 LARGE RIPE GREEN OR YELLOW PEAR, CUT INTO ⅓-INCH DICE

1 LARGE BANANA, CUT INTO ⅓-INCH DICE

½ TEASPOON VANILLA EXTRACT

1. Stir all the ingredients together in a medium bowl. Serve in small bowls with spoons.

BOOST IT: If you have leftover salad, store it in the fridge overnight and whip it into a smoothie the next morning. It's also excellent over plain yogurt.

ADAPT IT: Feel free to choose another favorite fruit to swap for any that don't suit your fancy.

MAKE AHEAD: Stir together the pineapple, mango, and kiwifruits the night before, cover, and store in the fridge overnight. In the morning, add the pear, banana, and vanilla up to 1 hour before serving.

·

BLACKBERRY ORANGE PUFFY PANCAKE

This is the sort of weekend breakfast that draws children into the kitchen to peek through the oven glass and watch the magic of baking at work. The batter rises into a golden puff crowned with an abundance of blackberries. It's just plain pretty, particularly with that little bit of sugar sprinkled over the top, which also adds a toothsome crust. No need to wait for berry season to make this, because frozen blackberries work like a dream. If you do use frozen blackberries, save the juices that drain off the berries as they thaw and stir them into your maple syrup.

2 TABLESPOONS SALTED BUTTER

4 EGGS

1 CUP WHOLE WHEAT PASTRY FLOUR, SPOONED AND LEVELED

1 CUP MILK

¼ CUP PURE MAPLE SYRUP

ZEST AND JUICE FROM ½ OF AN ORANGE

1 CUP BLACKBERRIES, FRESH OR FROZEN AND DEFROSTED

2 TABLESPOONS SUGAR

MAPLE SYRUP, TO SERVE (OPTIONAL)

1. Preheat the oven to 425°F.
2. Choose a 10-inch cast iron skillet or stainless steel skillet with an ovenproof handle. Lightly coat the pan with oil or nonstick cooking spray. Cut out a circle of parchment paper about 10 inches in diameter. Press the parchment into the pan so it adheres completely to the oiled bottom and sides. This will prevent sticking. Put the butter on top of the parchment and place the pan into the hot oven to melt the butter.

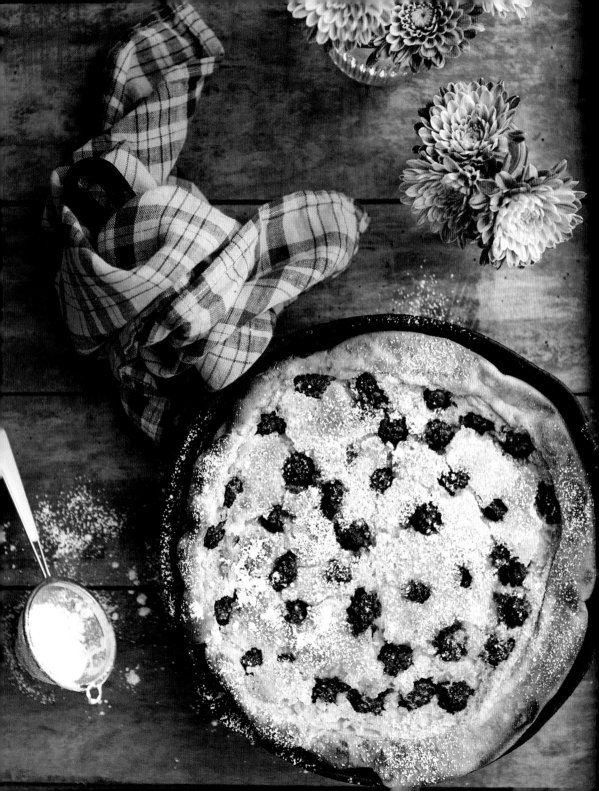

3. While the butter is melting, crack the eggs into the bowl of an electric mixer. Beat the eggs on high until pale yellow and a little foamy, about 1 minute. Add the whole wheat pastry flour, milk, maple syrup, orange zest, and 2 tablespoons of juice from the orange. Beat for 30 seconds, scraping down the sides as needed.

4. Remove the pan from the oven and swirl to coat the parchment paper with butter. Pour the batter into the pan. If using thawed frozen blackberries, drain off the juices and reserve. Gently scatter the blackberries evenly over the top of the batter. Sprinkle with the sugar and put into the oven.

5. Bake for about 20 minutes, until the pancake puffs, is golden brown, and is just firm to the touch in the center. Remove from the oven. The pancake will quickly deflate (don't worry, it will still be delicious).

6. Cut into wedges and serve immediately, either plain or with a light drizzle of maple syrup. If you have reserved blackberry juice, stir this into the maple syrup before serving.

BOOST IT: For a pretty finish, add a light dusting of confectioners' sugar just before serving.

BUCKWHEAT BLENDER CREPES

Making crepes in our house is as much a craft project as it is cooking. It's a toss-up as to what everyone's favorite part is: taking turns with the crepe pan or getting creative with the buffet of toppings. If you've never made crepes before, don't be intimidated. The batter is a breeze: everything goes into the blender at once. Learning to cook a proper crepe does involve some trial and error, but the payoff is worth the practice: golden, airy buckwheat crepes that pair just as well with ham and cheese as they do with fresh berries and confectioners' sugar.

3 EGGS

1 CUP MILK

½ CUP WATER

½ CUP BUCKWHEAT FLOUR, SPOONED AND LEVELED

½ CUP ALL-PURPOSE FLOUR, SPOONED AND LEVELED

¼ TEASPOON KOSHER SALT

2 TABLESPOONS SALTED BUTTER, MELTED

CREPE FIXINGS (SEE PAGE 193)

1. Put the eggs, milk, water, buckwheat flour, all-purpose flour, salt, and butter into the blender. Run on high for 30 seconds, stop to scrape down any flour stuck to the sides, then blend again for 30 seconds. Let the crepe batter rest at room temperature for at least 15 min-utes, ideally 1 hour. Allowing it to rest will save you some grief because the bubbles in the batter will fizzle out and your crepes will be less likely to tear.

2. When you are ready to make the crepes, set a 9- or 10-inch nonstick skillet or crepe pan over medium-high

heat. When the pan is hot, lightly brush the bottom and sides with oil or coat with nonstick cooking spray. Give the batter a gentle stir because the flour will have settled to the bottom. Pour ¼ cup of the batter into the pan, then lift the pan by the handle and quickly tilt to swirl the batter, coating the entire bottom and letting it travel up the sides a bit. Set the pan back down on the heat. Cook until the edges easily pull away from the pan and the crepe is barely brown. Wedge a spatula underneath and flip the crepe over. (If adding cheese or spinach—see opposite—do so now and cook until the cheese begins to soften or the spinach wilts, 30 seconds or so.)

Cook the second side until the bottom is lightly brown. Use a spatula to fold the crepe in half one way, and then in half again the other way, so it looks like a triangle.

3. Transfer the crepe to a plate and serve immediately with favorite fixings (see opposite). Continue making crepes as desired, lightly coating the pan with more oil as needed.

MAKE AHEAD: The batter is terrific made a day ahead, covered, and stored in the refrigerator. To store leftover crepes, leave them unfolded, wrap in plastic, and store in the refrigerator. They are great for a quick weekday breakfast. Just reheat in a skillet.

TIP

CREPE FIXINGS

Most of these toppings can be added after the crepes are cooked and plated; the exceptions are the cheese, ham, and spinach, which should be added onto the crepe as soon as it's flipped onto the second side, allowing the ingredients to warm before serving.

SWEET

Honey Stewed Summer Fruit (page 94)

A squeeze of lemon juice, a dab of butter, and a light shower of confectioners' sugar

A thin layer of chocolate hazelnut spread topped with fresh raspberries

A drizzle of maple syrup and a spoonful of chopped pecans

SAVORY

Diced leftover cooked vegetables (gently warmed)

Ratatouille (gently warmed)

Smoked salmon and sour cream

A few tablespoons of shredded Gruyère and a paper-thin slice of ham

A few tablespoons of shredded Cheddar and a small handful of spinach

3-INGREDIENT APPLE BUTTER TOASTER TARTS

Like a lot of families, sometimes we see weekends as a time for little indulgences that we forgo during the week—say, picking up croissants from a bakery on Saturday or giving the kids the green light to eat donuts after church on Sunday. My favorite kind of breakfast treats are the ones we make at home, and these apple toaster tarts are hard to top. It seems impossible that this crispy golden pastry can be made with just three ingredients. Thanks to store-bought puff pastry dough, it can. If you've never worked with premade puff pastry, you'll discover it's nothing short of magical, making even a baking amateur feel like a pro. So grab a kid (or two) and your rolling pin, and get busy. If you're lucky, you'll be able to stash a few leftover tarts to toast up on Monday morning.

1 LARGE GRANNY SMITH OR PINK LADY APPLE

1 SHEET (ABOUT 9 OUNCES) DEFROSTED PUFF PASTRY DOUGH (SEE NOTE)

½ CUP APPLE BUTTER, PREFERABLY WITHOUT ADDED SUGAR

SMALL DISH OF WATER

1. Preheat the oven to 400°F. Line a large baking sheet with parchment paper or a silicone baking mat.

2. Cut the apple off the core in 4 cuts. Lay the apple pieces flesh-side down on a cutting board and cut into very thin slices. It doesn't really matter what the slices look like, just be sure that they are quite thin. Set the apple slices aside.

3. Unwrap the puff pastry dough and unfold it. Lightly flour a work surface and a rolling pin and roll out the dough into a 12 × 16-inch rectangle. It will be very thin. Cut the dough into 16 rectangles that are 3 × 4 inches each. (If geome-

try isn't your strong suit, think of it like this: cut the rectangle of dough into quarters, then cut each quarter into quarters.)

4. Use a spatula to transfer 8 of the rectangles onto the prepared baking sheet, allowing space between them. Spoon 1 tablespoon of the apple butter onto the center of each rectangle and spread it to about ⅓-inch shy of the edge. Lay the apple slices on the apple butter, dividing them evenly among the 8 pieces of dough. Be sure to leave ¼ inch of space around the edge of the pastry. The apple slices can overlap.

5. Dab your finger into the water and lightly run it around the edge of one of the apple-covered pastries. Cover the pastry with one of the remaining 8 pieces of dough, lining up the edges on all sides. Use the tines of a fork to press the edges together to seal the apples inside, forming a little rectangular parcel. If a little apple butter sneaks out, just wipe it away and be sure the pastry appears sealed. Repeat with the remaining apple-covered pastries and rectangles of plain dough.

6. Bake for 20 to 22 minutes, until golden brown. Remove from the oven and serve when cool enough to handle.

Note: Puff pastry dough is sold in the freezer section of the market. Buy whole wheat dough if you can find it, and read the list of ingredients (some brands are better than others). Follow the directions on the package for defrosting.

MAKE AHEAD: Store tarts in a resealable bag or airtight container in the fridge for up to 3 days. They can also be stored in the freezer. Reheat in the toaster.

BIG JOE'S HUEVOS RANCHEROS

Big Joe was my father-in-law, a man with a larger-than-life personality, which is part of what earned him that nickname. Among his many passions was cooking, and these eggs were a signature dish. Thankfully, his recipe was passed down to the next generation, which means every Christmas morning my husband pulls it out and makes up a big pan for the family—a sort of gustatory homage to his dad. It's become my favorite meal of the holiday: soft eggs nestled in a smoky, chipotle-spiced tomato sauce under a cover of melted Cheddar. But don't wait for a special occasion to make it. It's neither fancy nor complicated, and it's so good you'll ask for seconds, which is exactly how Big Joe would have wanted it.

6 BACON SLICES

1 MEDIUM ONION, FINELY CHOPPED

ONE 28-OUNCE CAN DICED TOMATOES, WITH LIQUID

½ CUP WATER

1 CHIPOTLE CHILE EN ADOBO, MINCED INTO A PUREE (ABOUT 1 TABLESPOON)

1 TABLESPOON LIME JUICE

1 TEASPOON KOSHER SALT, PLUS A GENEROUS PINCH, DIVIDED

⅔ CUP ROUGHLY CHOPPED CILANTRO, DIVIDED

8 EGGS

8 CORN OR SMALL FLOUR TORTILLAS

1 CUP COARSELY GRATED SHARP CHEDDAR CHEESE

SLICED AVOCADO OR SOUR CREAM, FOR SERVING (OPTIONAL)

1. Set a large skillet over medium heat. Lay the bacon slices flat in the pan. Cook until the slices are deeply browned on one side and begin to curl up, about 5 minutes. Using a fork, turn the slices over and cook the second side until browned and most of the fat is rendered, another 3 minutes or so. Transfer to a plate covered with a couple of paper towels to absorb the drippings. When cool enough to handle, cut crosswise into ½-inch-wide pieces.

2. Pour off all but about 2 teaspoons of the bacon fat from the pan and return to medium heat. Add the onion and cook until tender and translucent, scraping up any tiny bacon bits off the bottom of the pan. Add the chopped bacon, tomatoes with their liquid, water, chipotle, lime juice, and 1 teaspoon of the salt to the pan. Stir well. Adjust the heat so the sauce simmers. Cook, stirring occasionally, until the tomatoes soften and a little of the liquid cooks off, about 10 minutes. It should look like a thick, chunky sauce. If it appears too dry, add 2 tablespoons more water.

3. Add half the cilantro and stir. Crack the eggs into the sauce, spacing them evenly in the pan, and sprinkle a generous pinch of salt over the top. Set a lid, large pot, or piece of aluminum foil over the skillet so that it's completely covered (I invert a wok on top of the pan). Simmer the eggs, adjusting the heat as needed, until done to your liking. For runny eggs, the whites should be cooked but the yolks still soft to the touch, about 6 to 8 minutes. Hard-cooked eggs will take an additional 2 minutes or so.

4. While the eggs are cooking, heat the tortillas in another skillet set over high heat or directly on the burner if you have a gas range, quickly warming each side. You want the tortillas warm and maybe a little blistered, but not crispy. Wrap in a napkin or dish towel to keep warm until ready to eat.

5. When the eggs are done, scatter the cheese and the remaining cilantro over the top. Serve right from the pan: spoon an egg and plenty of sauce onto a tortilla and top with avocado or sour cream, if desired. Eat like a very messy taco, or use a fork and knife.

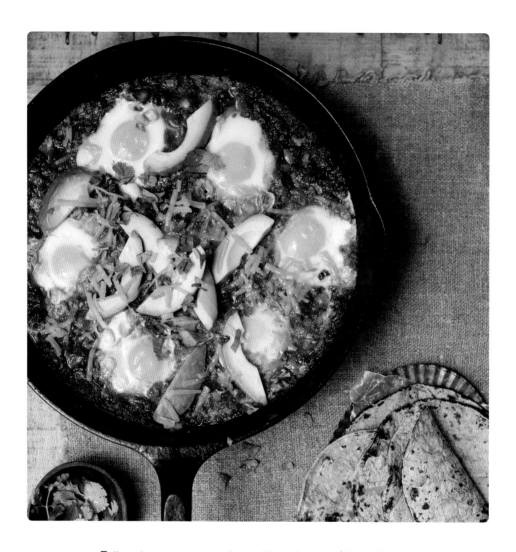

MAKE AHEAD: Follow the recipe just before adding the eggs (through the first addition of cilantro) and store the sauce in the fridge overnight. To prepare the dish the next day, re-heat the sauce, add the eggs, and continue the recipe. You may need to add a little more water when reheating. Leftovers keep well for up to 2 days.

ROASTED ROOT HASH WITH POACHED EGGS

My husband grew up on corned beef and hash, the kind that comes from a can and is traditionally topped with an egg. Although it's a dish he loves to this day, it's not one that suits my own cooking style, so I came up with this newfangled hash. A colorful mix of root vegetables gets tossed with a half-dozen seasonings and roasted in a hot oven, then finished with a couple of handfuls of peppery arugula and a splash of lemon juice. When you top it with a poached egg and the yolk breaks open over the vegetables? Well, it's pretty dreamy. If poaching eggs is outside your comfort zone, serve this with fried or boiled eggs instead.

1 LARGE SWEET POTATO (8 OUNCES)

2 OR 3 MEDIUM YUKON GOLD, YELLOW FINN, OR RED POTATOES (8 OUNCES)

1 LARGE PARSNIP (8 OUNCES), PEELED

3 MEDIUM CARROTS (8 OUNCES), PEELED

2 TABLESPOONS EXTRA-VIRGIN OLIVE OIL

1 ½ TEASPOONS SMOKED PAPRIKA

1 TEASPOON GROUND FENNEL

¼ TEASPOON GROUND CUMIN

1 TEASPOON GROUND CORIANDER

FEW DASHES OF CAYENNE

1 TEASPOON KOSHER SALT, PLUS MORE TO TASTE, IF DESIRED

1 LARGE YELLOW ONION, CUT INTO ¼-INCH-THICK HALF-MOON SLICES

2 LARGE HANDFULS ARUGULA

1 LEMON

2 TEASPOONS WHITE VINEGAR OR WHITE WINE VINEGAR

4 EGGS

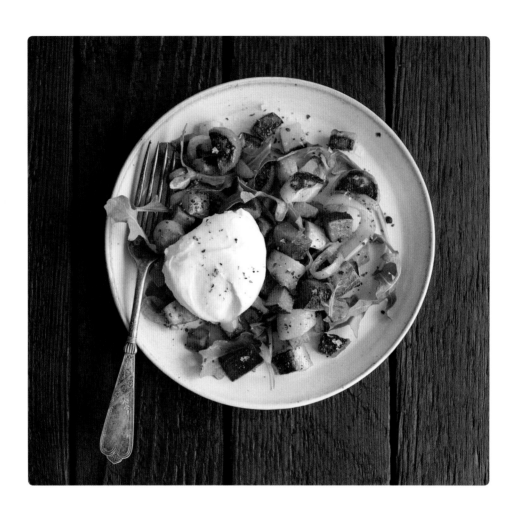

1. Preheat the oven to 425°F. Line 2 baking sheets with parchment paper or silicone baking mats.

2. Dice the sweet potato, potatoes, parsnip, and carrots into ½-inch pieces. Set aside.

3. In a large bowl, whisk together the olive oil, paprika, fennel, cumin, coriander, cayenne, and salt. Add the diced vegetables and onion to the bowl and toss well to coat. (I use my hands for this.) Distribute evenly over the prepared baking sheets. Don't wash the bowl yet!

4. Roast the vegetables for 30 to 35 minutes, until tender inside and a little crispy outside, stirring them halfway through. Transfer the vegetables back into the mixing bowl.

5. Add the arugula to the bowl. Cut the lemon in half and squeeze the juice over the vegetables. Stir well, taste, and add more salt if needed. Keep the vegetables in a warm spot near the stove while you poach the eggs.

6. Fill a 12-inch skillet with 2 to 3 inches of water. Add the vinegar, set over high heat, and bring to a boil. Once the water is boiling, lower the heat and let the water settle into a light simmer (little bubbles should appear across the bottom of the pan). Crack 1 of the eggs into a small ramekin and bring it close to the cooking water. Tip the egg gently into the simmering water in one fluid movement. Don't worry if it looks a little shaggy in the water. Repeat with the remaining 3 eggs in rapid succession, spacing them out in the pan until all 4 are simmering. Cook just until the whites look set, 2 to 3 minutes. For a firm yolk, cook an additional 1 to 2 minutes. You can check for doneness by lifting an egg with a slotted spoon and gently touching the center with your finger. Once cooked, use a slotted spoon to lift the eggs, one at a time, out of the water. Set each one on a dish towel briefly to absorb any water and transfer to a plate.

7. Divide the vegetables among 4 shallow bowls. Top each with a poached egg and a pinch of salt.

FARMERS' MARKET SALAD WITH WARM AND CRISPY GOAT CHEESE

It's Saturday morning, everyone is up, and the farmers' market is open. Go. Bring the kids. Peruse the stalls and find some lettuces that catch your eye. Look for vegetables to go along with the greens—juicy ripe tomatoes in summer or crisp bright fennel and radishes in winter. Add a bundle of fresh thyme. If you encounter a cheese maker, pick up some goat cheese. When you get home, unload everything, admire your wares, then get busy with this recipe. It's so good. Just ask the French, who have forever been pairing warm, bread-crumb-crusted goat cheese with delicate salads. *Bon appétit!*

6 OUNCES FRESH GOAT CHEESE (CHÈVRE)

⅓ CUP PANKO BREAD CRUMBS

¼ TEASPOON PLUS GENEROUS PINCH KOSHER SALT

2 TEASPOONS FINELY CHOPPED FRESH THYME

⅓ CUP PLUS 1 TEASPOON EXTRA-VIRGIN OLIVE OIL

4 GENEROUS HANDFULS OF SALAD GREENS, SUCH AS SPRING MIX OR MÂCHE,
OR 1 HEAD BUTTER LETTUCE, OR 4 HEADS LITTLE GEMS

2 SEASONAL VEGETABLES THAT YOU ENJOY RAW (ENOUGH TO GENEROUSLY GARNISH 4 SALADS),
SUCH AS TOMATOES, CUCUMBERS, FENNEL, RADISHES, OR CARROTS

2 TABLESPOONS WHITE WINE VINEGAR OR CHAMPAGNE VINEGAR

1 SMALL SHALLOT, MINCED

1 TEASPOON DIJON MUSTARD

1 TEASPOON HONEY

FRESHLY GROUND BLACK PEPPER

1. Preheat the oven to 400°F. Line a baking sheet with parchment paper.

2. Divide the goat cheese into 4 equal pieces and form into patties that are about 2½ inches in diameter. Stir together the bread crumbs, ¼ teaspoon of the salt, and the thyme in a small bowl.

3. Drizzle 1 teaspoon of the olive oil over the goat cheese and use your hands to spread it over the patties to coat. Place a patty into the bread crumb mixture, press down firmly to thoroughly cover one side of the cheese, turn it over, and press to coat the second side and edges. Place the patty on the prepared baking sheet. Repeat with the remaining cheese patties.

4. Bake for about 10 minutes, until lightly browned. Remove from the oven.

5. While the goat cheese bakes, make the salad and dressing. Wash the salad greens and dry well. Set aside. Prepare the seasonal vegetables as you like them in salad: cut tomatoes into wedges, slice cucumbers, shave fennel, cut carrots into diagonal slices, and so on. Set aside. To make the dressing, put the remaining ⅓ cup of olive oil and the vinegar, shallot, mustard, honey, generous pinch of salt, and several cracks of black pepper into a small jar. Screw on the lid and shake vigorously. Dribble a little dressing onto a lettuce leaf and taste. Adjust any ingredients, if needed.

6. To assemble the salad, put the salad greens into a large bowl and toss with a small amount of the vinaigrette. Taste, and add more dressing if desired. Divide the greens among 4 plates. Lay the seasonal vegetables along one side of the greens, dividing them among the plates, and drizzle a little dressing on top (you may have leftover dressing, which will keep in the fridge for a few days). Use a spatula to gently transfer the goat cheese patties from the baking sheet onto the plated greens. Serve.

ACKNOWLEDGMENTS

"*I get to do this for a job?*" It's a rhetorical question I find myself asking out loud and often, sometimes to friends, occasionally just to myself, as I putter around my kitchen, scribble in a battered notebook, tinker with ingredients, taste and ask everyone around me to taste, and put it all down on the laptop in my tiny home office. I'm so grateful that this is what I call work. I'm even more thankful for the many folks who care about and support what I do.

On the professional front, I frequently think about the smart women I have to lean on, collaborate with, and look to for inspiration. A special shout-out to my community of registered dietitians, most especially Sally Kuzemchak and Maryann Jacobsen, who lent their professional expertise to the pages of this book. To Courtney Woo, who was a gift to have in my kitchen during her dietetic internship. To the writers who make me want to be a better writer: Sarah Copeland, Cheryl Sternman Rule, Andrea Nguyen, Phyllis Grant, and Emma Christensen. And to Pam Hommeyer, who proofread my manuscript so meticulously, she made me look like a far better grammarian than I really am.

This book wouldn't be what it is without the eye and heart of photographer Erin Scott, who made this not just a job but a creative journey. Her thoughtfulness, aesthetic, and gentle energy couldn't have been more perfect for me or my recipes. And thank you to food stylist Lillian Kang, a total delight who knocked it out of the park on the pretty front. Thank you also to Leigh Oshirak for being such a great sounding board and supportive friend.

Recipe testers, I hope you have a smidge of an idea how enormously important you are: Mary Ellen Stumpfl, Heather Wall, Lily Daniel, Jane McKay, Kate Banfield, Lucy Dendinger, Kendra Prime, Heather Prime, Charlotte Prime, Pam Hochman, and Claire Bobrow. Extra-special thanks to Sarah Stadlin, who recipe tested like a total professional; Spring Utting, whose joy and energy are unparalleled; and Pam Rupright, whom I trust with my cornmeal muffins as much as with my kids.

What would I do without you, Carole Bidnick? You are the fairy godmother of literary agents. Thanks for finding *Rise and Shine* such a sweet and perfect home. And to everyone at Roost Books, especially my editor, Jennifer Urban-Brown, who seemed to embrace this project wholeheartedly from day one and gave me room to make it my own.

Giant hugs of gratitude to my nears and dears for their love, wisdom, and enthusiasm: my mom, who sets the standard for nourishing a family in every way; my dad, whose approval means as much to me today as it did when I was ten; my brother Mark and his beloved, Alison, both chefs, who are always at the other end of the line when I have a cooking 911; and to Annie, Maureen, Meagan, Kristin, and Dave (invoke the megaphone): THANK YOU!

I am enormously blessed to have such a wonderful tribe of girlfriends—amazing women, every one. I hope you know how much your support matters. And to my extended family of blog readers at *Mom's Kitchen Handbook:* You were at the forefront of my mind as I developed every one of these recipes. May they bring nourishment, ease, and inspiration to your mornings.

Finally (and for this, picture me shouting from the top of the butcher block in the center of my kitchen), I want to thank my husband, Joe, who eats my food with the eagerness of a teenage boy, listens to me rattle on about nutrition as if it's the first time he's ever heard it, and edits my work with the attention of a Google intern. Thank you to my three girls, Isabelle, Rosie, and Virginia, for always giving it to me straight and for facing every plate of eggs and stack of waffles these past months—whether for breakfast, lunch, or dinner—with patience and enthusiasm. I love cooking for and with you all.

RESOURCES

ONLINE

American Egg Board, Egg Nutrition Center (www
.eggnutritioncenter.org)

Center for Urban Education about Sustainable
Agriculture (www.cuesa.org)

Environmental Working Group (www.ewg.org)

"EWG's Food Scores" (www.ewg.org/foodscores)

Fooducate (www.fooducate.com)

King Arthur Flour (www.kingarthurflour.com)

The Kitchn (www.thekitchn.com)

Real Mom Nutrition blog, Sally Kuzemchak, MS,
RD (www.realmomnutrition.com)

U.S. Department of Agriculture, USDA National
Nutrient Database for Standard Reference
(http://ndb.nal.usda.gov)

U.S. Department of Health and Human
Services (HHS) and U.S. Department of
Agriculture, "Dietary Guidelines for Amer-
icans" (www.health.gov/dietaryguidelines)

BOOKS

Jill Castle and Maryann Jacobsen, MS, RD, *Fear-
less Feeding: How to Raise Healthy Eaters from
High Chair to High School* (Jossey-Bass, 2013)

Victoria Shanta Retelny, with Jovanka JoAnn
Milivojevic, *The Essential Guide to Healthy
Healing Foods* (Alpha, 2011)

Cheryl Sternman Rule, *Yogurt Culture: A Global
Look at How to Make, Bake, Sip, and Chill the
World's Creamiest, Healthiest Food* (Hough-
ton Mifflin Harcourt, 2015)

OTHER RESOURCES

Dwyer, J. "Defining Nutritious Breakfasts and
Their Benefits." *Journal of the Academy of Nutrition and Dietetics* 2014 (Suppl. 3): S5–S7.

O'Neil, C., C. Byrd-Bredbenner, D. Hayes, L.
Jana, S. Klinger, and S. Stephenson-Martin.
"The Role of Breakfast in Health: Definition
and Criteria for a Quality Breakfast." *Journal
of the Academy of Nutrition and Dietetics*
2014 (Suppl. 3): S8–S26.

Wansink, B., D. R. Just, C. R. Payne, and M.
Klinger. "Attractive Names Sustain Increased
Vegetable Intake in Schools." *Preventive Med-
icine* 2012 (55, no. 4): 330–32.

Widenhorn-Muller, K., K. Hille, and J. Klenk.
"Influence of Having Breakfast on Cognitive
Performance and Mood in 13- to 20-Year-Old
High School Students: Results of a Crossover
Trial." *Pediatrics* 2008 (1222, no. 2): 279–84.

INDEX

Roost Books
An imprint of Shambhala Publications, Inc.
4720 Walnut Street
Boulder, Colorado 80301
roostbooks.com

Printed in China

♾This edition is printed on acid-free paper that meets
the American National Standards Institute Z39.48 Standard.
♻Shambhala Publications makes every effort to print on recycled paper.
For more information please visit www.shambhala.com.

Distributed in the United States by Penguin Random House LLC
and in Canada by Random House of Canada Ltd

Designed by Daniel Urban-Brown

LIBRARY OF CONGRESS CATALOGING-IN-PUBLICATION DATA

Morford, Katie Sullivan, author.
Rise and shine: better breakfasts for busy mornings/Katie Sullivan Morford.
      pages   cm
Includes index.
ISBN 978-1-61180-294-8 (pbk.: alk. paper)
1. Breakfasts. I. Title.
TX733.M667 2016
641.5′2—dc23
2015026645